Psychosis - Phenomenology, Psychopathology and Pathophysiology

Edited by Kenjiro Fukao

Published in London, United Kingdom

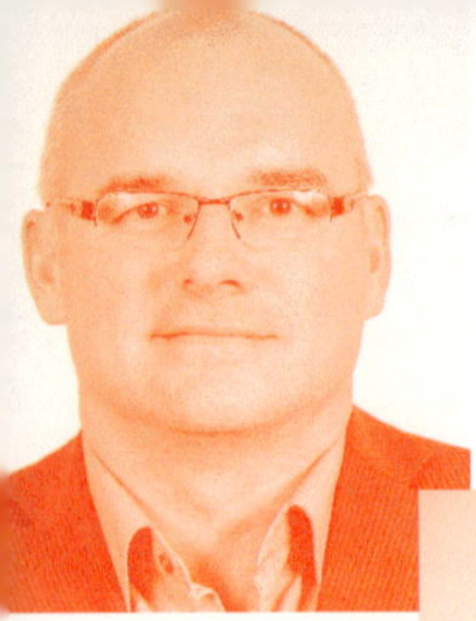
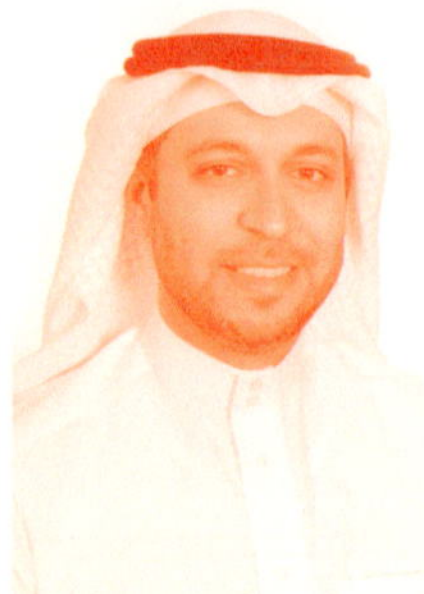
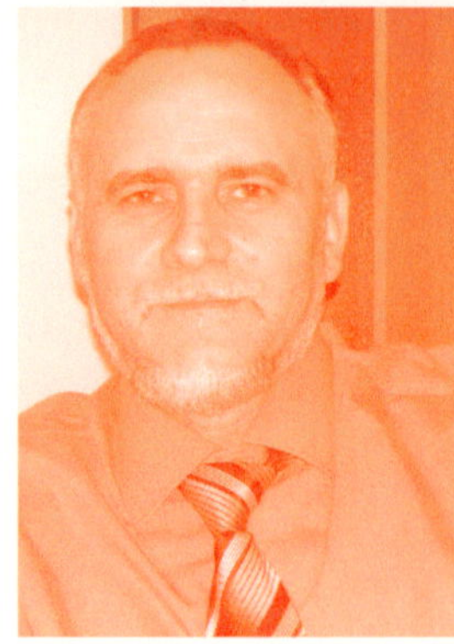
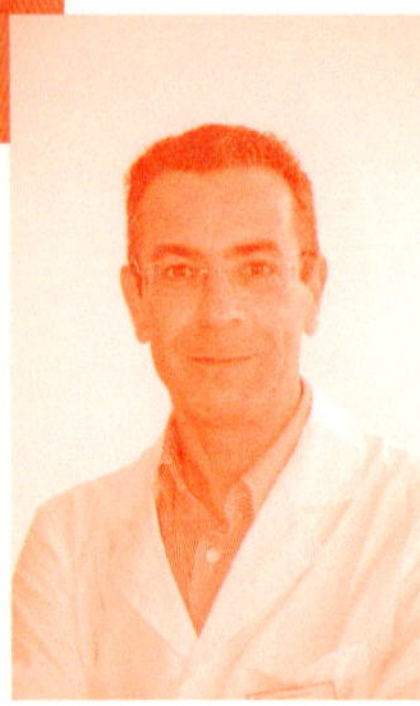
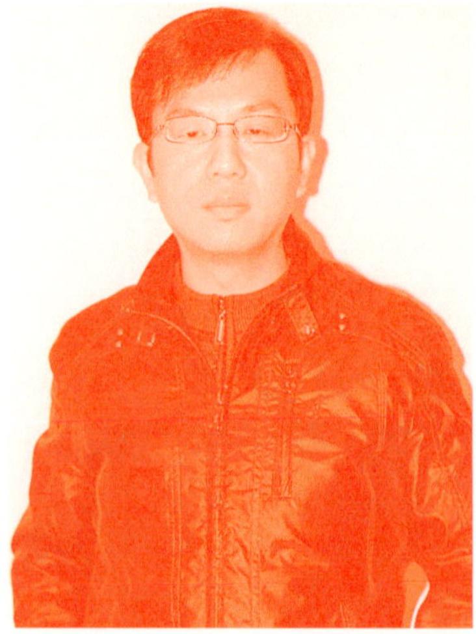
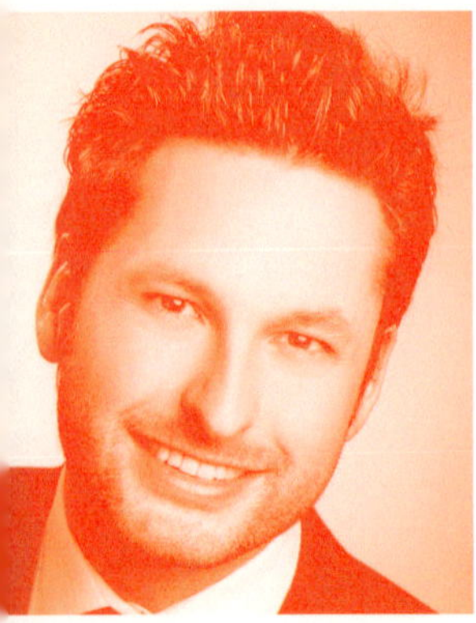
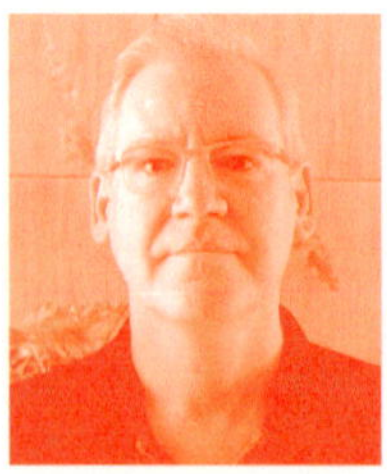

IntechOpen

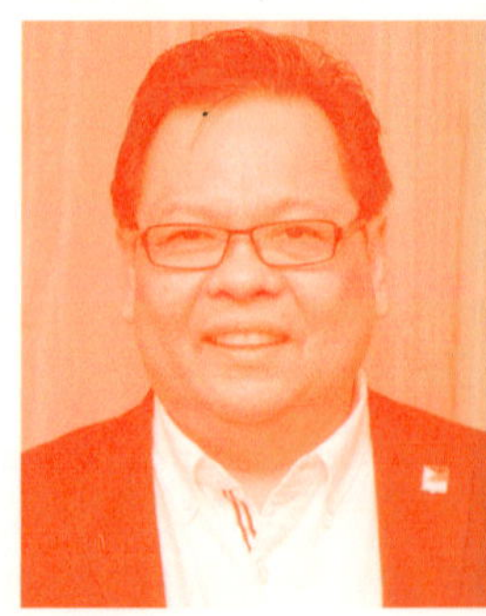
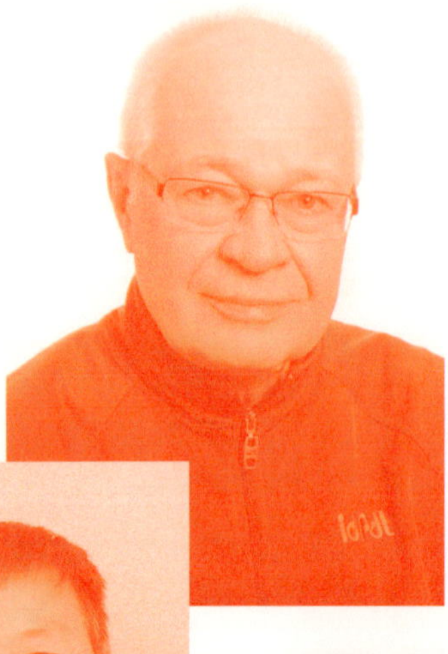
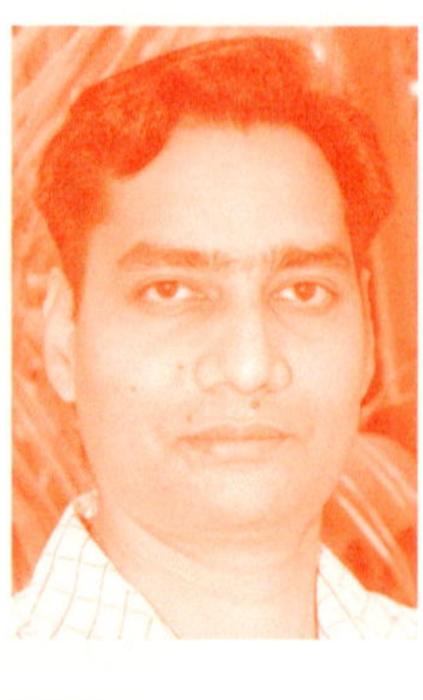
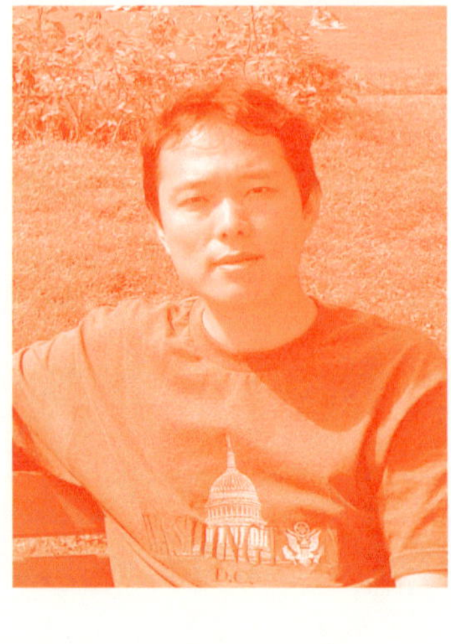
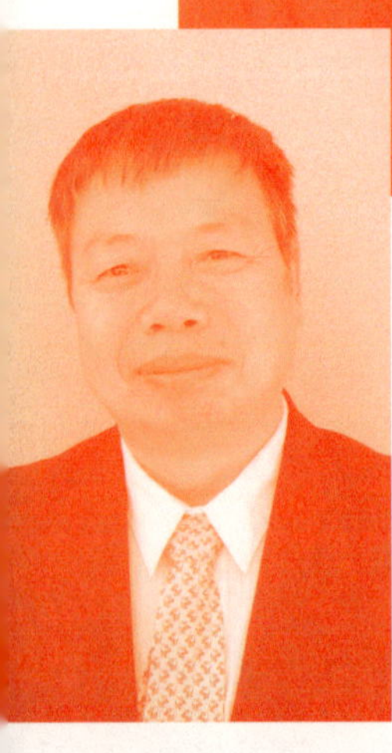
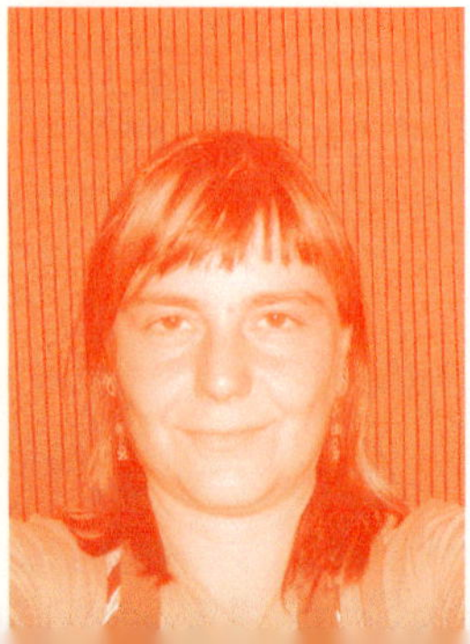

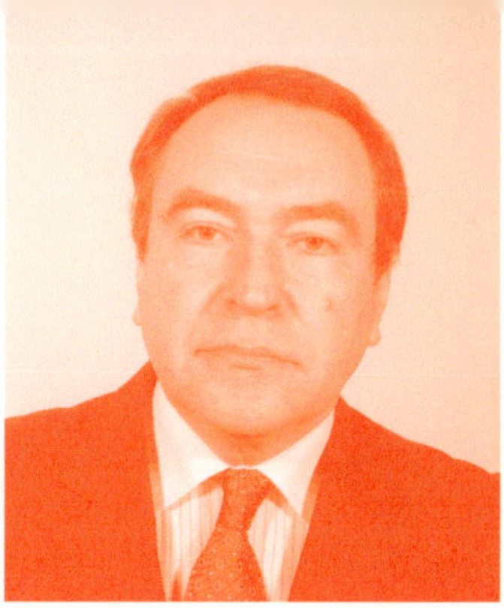
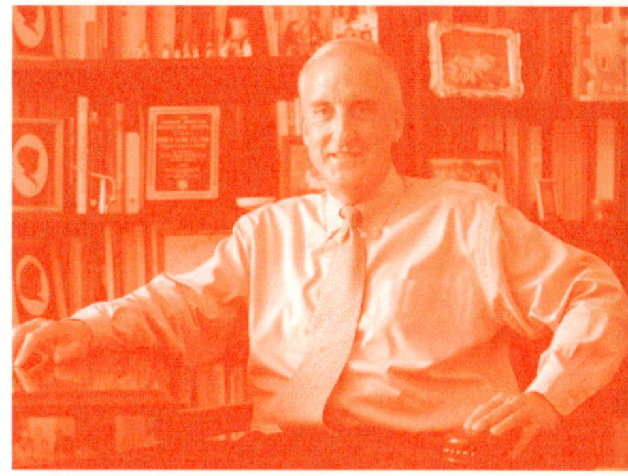
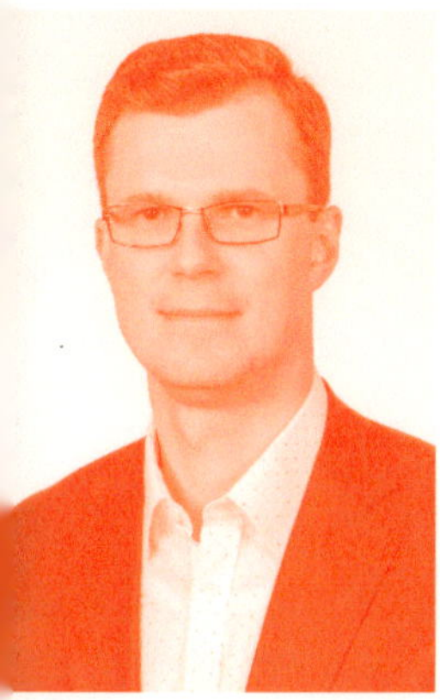
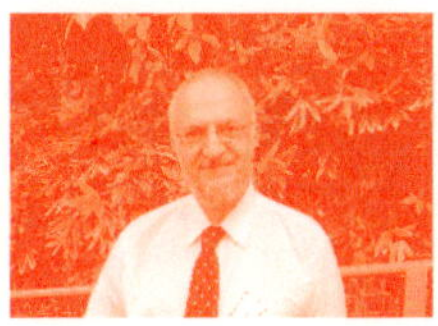
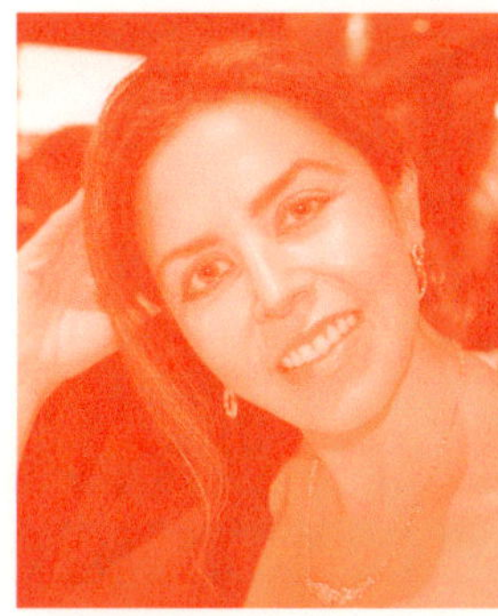

Supporting open minds since 2005

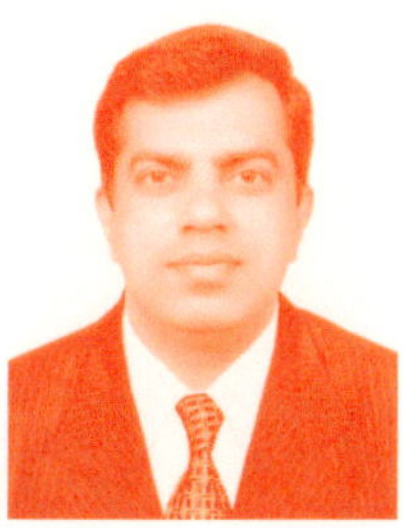
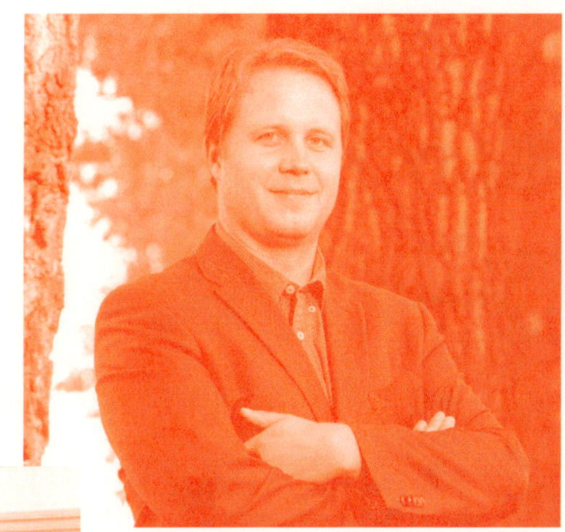
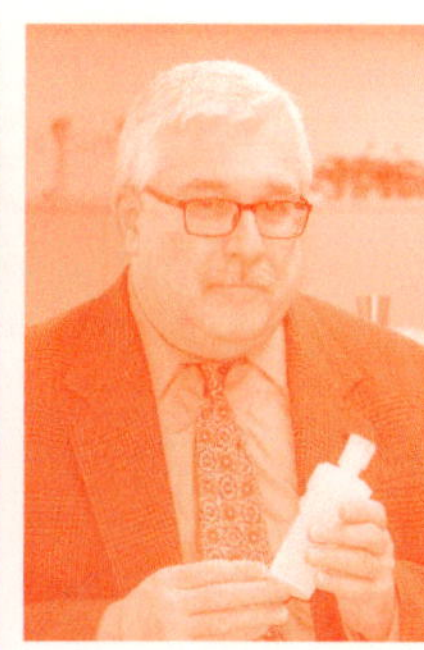
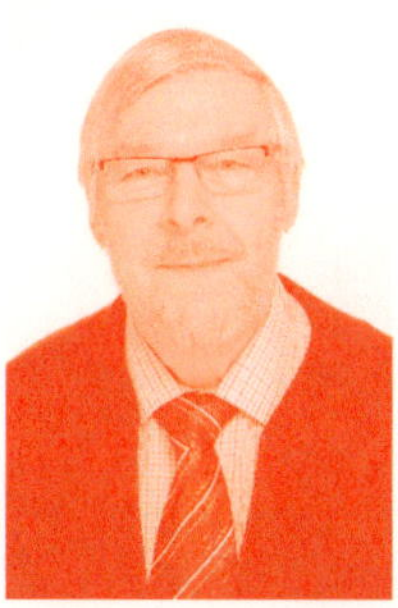
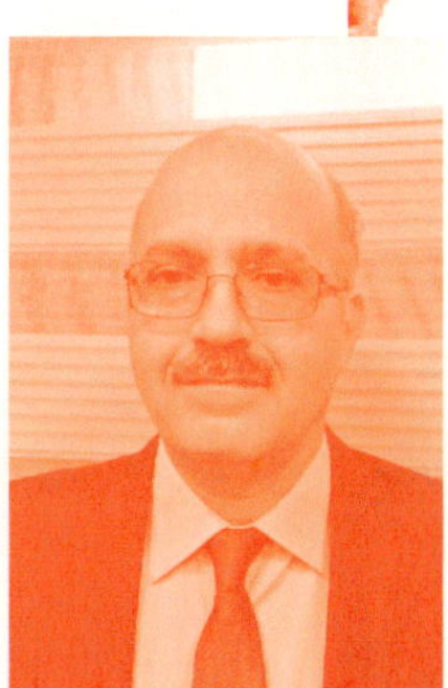
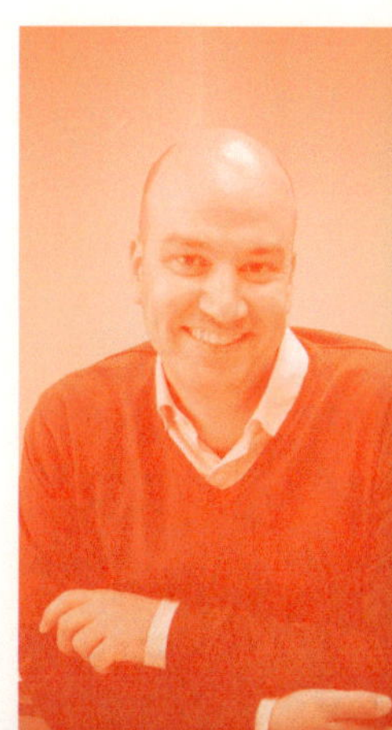
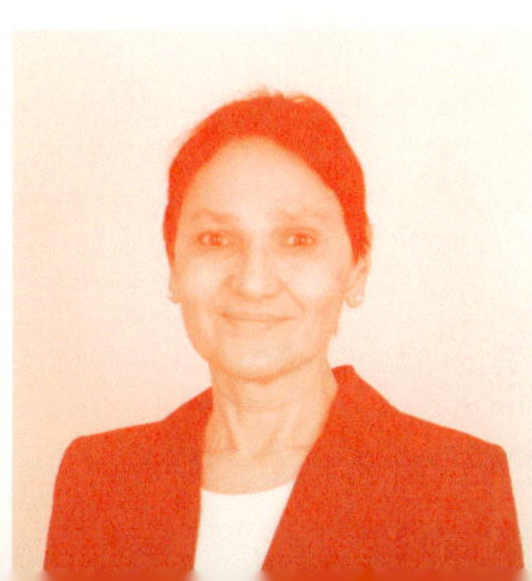

Psychosis - Phenomenology, Psychopathology and Pathophysiology
http://dx.doi.org/10.5772/intechopen.77646
Edited by Kenjiro Fukao

Contributors
Wafa Abdelghaffar, Oussama Sidhom, Rym Rafrafi, Lilia Laadhar, Adolfo J. Cangas, Francisco Martin-Murcia, Esmaeil Shahsavand Ananloo, Zsófia Borbála Dombi, Agota Barabassy, Barbara Sebe, István Laszlovszky, György Németh, Kommu Naga Mohan, Pranay Amruth Maroju, Mihaela Fadgyas Stanculete, Octavia Capatina, Kenjiro Fukao

First published in London, United Kingdom, 2022 by IntechOpen
IntechOpen is the global imprint of INTECHOPEN LIMITED, registered in England and Wales, registration number: 11086078, 5 Princes Gate Court, London, SW7 2QJ, United Kingdom
Printed in Croatia

British Library Cataloguing-in-Publication Data
A catalogue record for this book is available from the British Library

Additional hard and PDF copies can be obtained from orders@intechopen.com

Psychosis - Phenomenology, Psychopathology and Pathophysiology
Edited by Kenjiro Fukao
p. cm.
Print ISBN 978-1-83969-044-0
Online ISBN 978-1-83969-045-7
eBook (PDF) ISBN 978-1-83969-046-4

For EU product safety concerns:
IN TECH d.o.o., Prolaz Marije Krucifikse Kozulić 3, 51000 Rijeka, Croatia, info@intechopen.com or visit our website at intechopen.com.

Meet the editor

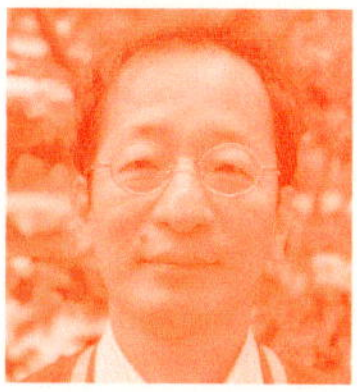

Kenjiro Fukao, MD, Ph.D. graduated from Kyoto University School of Medicine and majored in psychiatry. Then he specialized in psychiatric epileptology, working in the National Epilepsy Center in Shizuoka, Japan, University Hospital of Zürich, Switzerland and Kyoto University Hospital. He subsequently specialized in psychiatric epileptology, working at the National Epilepsy Center, Shizuoka, Japan, and the University Hospital of Zürich, Switzerland. He obtained a Ph.D. with research on the magnetoencephalographic study of patients with epileptic psychosis. He trained in phenomenological psychopathology with anthropological psychiatrist Prof. Kimura Bin. Currently, Dr. Fukao is a professor in the Department of Psychology, Faculty of Human Sciences, Tezukayama Gakuin University, Japan.

Contents

Preface

Psychosis has historically been the central problem of psychiatry because it harms both reason and emotion, even sometimes personality itself, and, whether rapidly or gradually, destroys the productive life of people. It is also intriguing for researchers due to the variety of subjective symptoms, which are enigmatic and provoke artistic imaginations.

Schizophrenia, the representative syndrome of psychotic disorders, still remains the hardest subject for psychiatric practice, although recently said to be becoming milder in the clinical features. Pathogenesis of schizophrenia is not yet solved and thus antipsychotic medications are not curative but rather symptomatic therapies.

This volume presents current research for the elucidation of psychosis in three different aspects: phenomenological, which relates to the philosophical or conceptual basis of psychosis; psychopathological, which relates to clinical manifestations of psychosis; and pathophysiological, which relates to the scientific pursuit for the mechanism of psychosis.

Chapter 1, "Understanding / Psychosis," deals with the very basis of diagnosis of psychosis differentiated from neurosis or psychogenic symptoms, namely, un-understandability as the impossibility of understanding in Japers' sense.

Chapter 2, "The Axiological Structure in Psychosis," presents the phenomenological-existential analysis of psychosis and suggests its therapeutic implications.

Chapter 3, "Clinical Staging in Schizophrenia Spectrum Disorders," summarizes the state-of-the-art knowledge of clinical staging in schizophrenia spectrum disorders.

Chapter 4, "The Many Faces of Negative Symptoms in Schizophrenia," addresses recent advances regarding the concepts, definitions, and classifications of negative symptoms of schizophrenia and their etiological model.

Chapter 5, "Role of Immunity in Pathogenesis of Psychosis," reviews the immune-inflammatory theory of schizophrenia and its clinical implications.

Chapter 6, "The Role of Epigenetics in Psychosis," deals with the possible significance of epigenetic dysregulation in the pathogenesis of schizophrenia.

Finally, Chapter 7, "DNA Methyltransferases and Schizophrenia: Current Status," reviews the dysregulation of DNA methyltransferases in schizophrenia.

This book provides readers with novel insight into psychosis and will help to advance research in the field.

Kenjiro Fukao, M.D., Ph.D.
Tezukayama Gakuin University,
Osaka, Japan

Section 1

Phenomenology

Chapter 1

Understanding / Psychosis

Kenjiro Fukao

Abstract

"Understanding" in Jaspers' sense is the essential concept for defining psychosis, although its relationship is paradoxical, that is, psychosis is defined by un-understandability or inability to understand. Un-understandability means the inability of empathizing with the patient's mind and implies the existence of a pathological process in the patient's brain. The pivotal concept which makes psychotic patients be judged as irresponsible in forensic cases is disturbed self-understanding or un-understandability of their own intentions. It is suggested that self-disorder representing psychosis might be based on disturbed self-understanding.

Keywords: psychosis, understanding, un-understandability, Jaspers, self-understanding

1. Introduction

"Understanding psychosis" is in itself a contradictory remark, because psychosis is defined as an "un-understandable" entity. As is well-known, "understanding" in classic psychopathology has a special meaning which differentiates psychosis from neurosis defined as psychogenic symptoms. As neurotic symptoms like anxiety or phobia are "understandable", that is, imaginable and relivable on the basis of normal mental life, they can be thought of as quantitative extremes of normal mental activities, and therefore can be treated psychologically. In contrast, psychotic symptoms like hallucinations or delusions are qualitatively different from normal mental activities and cannot be imagined as their quantitative extremes. This qualitative difference should be considered as a marker of the existence of pathological processes in the patient's brain.

While nowadays various neurotic disorders which had been considered as psychogenic have turned to be thought to have some neural basis, psychotic symptoms still remain a special group of symptoms, which indicate difficulty for purely psychological treatments. Therefore, "understanding" still remains an important clinical methodology, although it is entirely subjective and fairly ambiguous. This chapter reviews and examines the implications and possibilities of the concept of "understanding" for clarifying what is psychosis.

2. Understanding and Jaspers

The concept of understanding in the specialized sense is introduced in psychiatry by Karl Theodor Jaspers (1883–1969), who was a German psychiatrist and later an existential philosopher, but it is not he who invented it. This methodological concept was introduced in order to distinguish the method of history from that of natural sciences by German historian Johann Gustav Bernhard Droysen (1808–1884). Then German philosopher Wilhelm Christian Ludwig Dilthey (1833–1911) adapted it from history to psychology. Dilthey endeavored to establish a methodological basis of human sciences (*Geisteswissenschaften* in German) and proposed understanding (*Verstehen*) as the distinct and essential methodology of them, opposed to explanation (*Erklären*) characteristic of natural sciences. Understanding is a subjective method based on empathy and imagination, contrasted with that explanation is an objective method based on some theory or logical interpretation.

Because psychiatry is not a pure natural science like other disciplines of medicine, but an interdisciplinary field comprising natural, human and social sciences, it was reasonable that Jaspers adopted understanding as a principal method of psychiatry, besides causal explanation. In the monumental textbook "General Psychopathology (*Allgemeine Psychopathologie*)" [1, 2] (abbreviated as GP in the following), he urged psychiatrists to consider the difference between psychical symptoms and somatic symptoms, that is, the former is subjective and the latter is basically objective. Causal explanation can only be applied to objective phenomena and so-called "psychological explanation" should exactly be called understanding as far as it is purely subjective.

At the time Jaspers published the first edition of GP in 1913, he was facing and had to oppose the then propagating influence of psychoanalysis. He pointed out the methodological weakness of psychoanalysis in various ways and characterized it as "pseudo-understanding" or "as-if-understanding (*Als-ob-Verstehen*)" in which plausible but fictitious interpretation is mistaken for understanding (GP, pp. 306–7).

It is important to note that Jaspers also emphasized the limitation of understanding. He writes, it is not that the psyche can only be understood and cannot be causally explained, but it can also be explained. While explanation has no limits, as it continues to widen the range in proportion to the progress of neuroscience, "with understanding there are limits everywhere" (GP, p. 305), as it is only based on our innate ability of empathy and imagination. Also, he writes, "Understanding by itself does not lead to any causal explanation except in indirect fashion when it happens to come up against the un-understandable" (GP, p. 305). In other words, understanding indicates the existence of a pathological process in the human psyche not by its ability but by its inability. This is the seemingly paradoxical feature that makes the concept of understanding look somewhat confusing, but also makes it unreplaceable by any other concepts.

3. Psychosis as the un-understandable

There are common misunderstandings of Jaspers' characterization of psychotic disorders as the "un-understandable". Some clinicians take un-understandability for disorder of communication often seen in chronic cases of schizophrenia. As such cases often show thought disorder in which logical and verbal rules appear disrupted, resulting in difficulty of communication with others, the expression "schizophrenia is un-understandable" might often be misunderstood as describing such a situation. However, the right meaning of "schizophrenia is un-understandable" is that psychic phenomena characteristic of schizophrenia cannot be imagined and relived by healthy people. "Understanding" of Jaspers' meaning is not at all related to logical or verbal thinking.

Another misunderstanding of the un-understandability of psychosis is that it is taken for indicating the impossibility of scientific elucidation of psychosis or schizophrenia. Whereas Jaspers was critical about the premature adoption of the biological explanation of psychotic disorders, accusing such attempts as "brain mythologies" (GP, p. 18), he did not deny the possibility of the future success of such scientific research for the cause of psychosis in the brain. In fact, his characterization of psychosis as the un-understandable implies the necessity of biological research, because when understanding faces limitations, he writes, "each limitation is a fresh stimulus to formulate the problem of cause anew" (GP, p. 305). Jaspers believed that schizophrenia should have some biological cause, which is gradually appearing as un-understandable symptoms and eventually bringing the person into a sterile deficient state.

Psychosis in the meaning of Japers is not confined to schizophrenia. It includes mood disorders, although in the classical definition of the cyclic appearing of severe affective symptoms. While the diagnostic criteria of mood disorders have been significantly broadened since his era, resulting in the inclusion of people without any psychotic nature, Jaspers' definition of mood disorder was much narrower, confined to severe depression (melancholy) and bipolar disorders (manic depressive illness). He characterized it as psychosis, not because of the existence of hallucinations or delusions like modern operational diagnostic systems, but because of un-understandability in the same meaning as schizophrenia.

What is, however, the sameness between schizophrenia and severe mood disorder, if it is not the existence of hallucinations or delusions which are un-understandable symptoms? It might be said that those two have disorders in reality testing in common from the behavioral viewpoint. While, from Jaspers' viewpoint of understanding, because the experience of mood disorders is fairly understandable on the basis of normal affective life, it seems to differ from schizophrenic experience that is un-understandable. Un-understandability of mood disorders exists not in the mood itself, but in its manner of appearance. That is, affective symptoms in mood disorders appear cyclically with a certain period like automatic machinery, almost not at all related to incidents in mental life. Patients feel sad or cheerful for a certain duration without any incidents that are understandable by others to induce those affects. This is the meaning of un-understandability of mood disorders.

The two major types of psychosis, schizophrenia and mood disorders are thus defined as the "un-understandable". Then another question might arise: why there are only two types in psychosis? The author's answer is based on Kraepelin's principle of dichotomy, that is, disease process without regard to pathogenesis could only be classified into two forms, chronic-progressive and acute-recurrent. In addition, the chronic-progressive process implies gradual diffusion and the acute-recurrent process does localized irritation. Therefore psychosis also should be classified almost necessarily into two corresponding forms, chronic-diffuse and acute-local, whose actualizations are schizophrenia and mood disorders respectively. Thus the "un-understandable" manifests itself as gradually permeative in schizophrenia, whereas in mood disorders it does as mechanically cyclic.

4. Psychosis, responsibility, and self-understanding

One reason, and the most important one from the sociocultural viewpoint, why the psychopathological distinction between psychosis and various psychogenic states should be defined is that it matters forensic judgments on responsibility for illegal acts. A person afflicted with the severe psychotic disorder would not be punished because of a lack of responsibility for illegal acts, which are supposed to have been executed by lack of reason resulting from the disorder.

Here it is to be clarified what is lack of reason because the meaning of the word "reason" is quite ambiguous. Concretely, it can be classified into three categories.

The first is the insufficiency of the ability for distinguishing right from wrong, which is represented by people with intellectual disabilities or dementia virtually equated with children. The second is acute confusion with impairment of consciousness, which can be induced by intoxication by alcohol or other psychotropic substances, and also by epileptic disorders. In principle, memories of the behavior are disturbed in these cases. The third category is the most complicated cases, namely, people with schizophrenia or delusional disorders, who are with sufficient ability for telling right and wrong, and without any impairment of consciousness.

Then, what is the reason why people with schizophrenia or delusional disorders are thought "without reason"? It is because their delusions are, although often wrong in content, never correctable by any factual evidence or sincere persuasion. In other words, the patients lack the ability of "reality testing", as they take their delusions as more real than the reality shared by others intersubjectively.

However, an important question remains: what is the difference between the delusions of the patients and queer thoughts held by, for example, religious minorities? Is it that whereas a psychotic delusion is held only by a patient, a religious belief is held by, however small it is, a collective? However, this question is ultimately insoluble, because there is always a possibility of the existence of co-believers of the thought, especially in the contemporary setting in which queer religious and other kinds of thoughts are scattered and pervading through the internet without forming any physical collective.

It is, therefore, necessary to define the essential deficit of the patients with psychotic delusions, which justifies the lack of responsibility, without being based on the content of the belief. The concept of understanding is here again useful as shown in the following.

Let us think about a typical legal case of a person with schizophrenia. He committed a kind of crime, for example, violence against a woman. He accepts that it is a fact that he executed brute force on her, but he does not accept that it was directed by his intention. He does not mean that it was an accident or a mistake, and he has a clear memory about the violence he employed. What he insists is that whereas the violence was executed by his body, it was directed by another person's intention, that is, the agent of his body was not himself at that time. It is a quite irrational statement, which describes an un-understandable experience that we, the psychically healthy, cannot relive or imagine.

The reason why delusional patients should be thought irresponsible is, however, not the fact itself that their experience during the criminal acts is un-understandable by the healthy people. If it was the reason, it would be in effect the same situation as the queer thoughts held by the minorities. The true reason is the fact that the patient himself cannot understand his own intention. Our voluntary acts are based on our intentions and the connection between our intentions and our acts is always understandable without any verification, which is the basic fact for the responsibility. In the psyche of people with schizophrenia, however, the connection is broken and becomes un-understandable, so that the agent of his acts is lost and found in another, often undesired horrible person. Therefore the patient was himself horrified when he executed the violence. In this way, the un-understandability of the insistence of people with psychotic disorders stems from the un-understandability of their own intentions, so to speak, a disorder of self-understanding.

5. Self-understanding as the basis of self-disorder

Disorder of self-understanding has much broader significance than that has within the range of forensic psychiatry. With regard to general psychopathology of schizophrenia or psychosis, it could be thought to constitute the basis of various "bizarre" hallucinations and delusions, generally called ego disorder (*Ich-Störung*) or self-disorder, for example, verbal hallucinations criticizing or commenting on the patient, passivity phenomena and delusion of observation. Although Jaspers characterized schizophrenia as the un-understandable and therefore incomprehensible, it seems rather consistently comprehensible from the viewpoint of self-disorder, as once Kurt Schneider (1887–1967) and lately phenomenological psychopathologists have maintained [3–5].

Whereas the self is what should be the most understandable for us, because it is the very basis of the understandability of the world which we live in, nevertheless, it becomes un-understandable for the patients with schizophrenia. When the self is un-understandable, all the percepts coming in from the outside or even from inside the body become mysterious and alienated, resulting in the entire world being opaque and un-understandable. Furthermore, they cannot effectively respond to and resist the situation, because their own intention also becomes alienated, remaining their bodies impotent and paralyzed. Thus various bizarre and un-understandable complaints and disorganized behaviors that the patients show are to be comprehended as manifestations of the predicament into which they are being fallen and their desperate striving against it.

6. Summary

Modern operational diagnostic system like DSM-5 lacks the essential concept for defining psychosis [6]. Understanding and un-understandability are, although somewhat confusing because of the paradoxical feature, and too ambiguous from the viewpoint of operationalization, still necessary concepts for psychiatrists to make clinical practice effectively. Also, there seems to be a need for the development of the concept of self-understanding, based on that of understanding, for deeper comprehension and more sensible treatments of psychotic patients.

Author details

Kenjiro Fukao
Faculty of Human Science, Department of Psychology, Tezukayama Gakuin University, Japan

*Address all correspondence to: fukao@tezuka-gu.ac.jp

References

[1] Jaspers K. Allgemene Psychopathologie. Fünfte unveränderte Auflage. Berlin Heidelberg GmbH: Springer-Verlag; 1948

[2] Jaspers K (Hoenig J, Hamilton MW, trans.). General Psychopathology. Baltimore: Johns Hopkins University Press; 1997

[3] Schneider K (Hamilton MW, trans.). Clinical Psychopathology. Oxford: Grune & Stratton; 1959

[4] Parnas J, Handest P. Phenomenology of anomalous self-experience in early schizophrenia. Comprehensive Psychiatry. 2003;**44**(2):121-134

[5] Fuchs T. The self in schizophrenia: Jaspers, Schneider, and beyond. In: Stangellini G, Fuchs T, editors. One Century of Karl Jaspers' General Psychopathology. Oxford: Oxford University Press; 2013. pp. 245-257

[6] Parnas J. On psychosis: Karl Jaspers and beyond. In: Stangellini G, Fuchs T, editors. One Century of Karl Jaspers' General Psychopathology. Oxford: Oxford University Press; 2013. pp. 208-228

Chapter 2

The Axiological Structure in Psychosis

Francisco Martín-Murcia and Adolfo J. Cangas

Abstract

In this chapter the value structure will be described as one of the essential existential foundations from a phenomenological perspective. Psychosis could be understood as the result of structural modifications of the self in anchoring the lifeworld. These modifications would mainly be due to failure in the construction of intersubjectivity and therefore of the common sense or basic intuitive tuning of the social world. This failure precisely involves the axiological component of psychotic being-in-the-world, so its description will be emphasized, along with its peculiarities and similarities to other ways of functioning of this axis of values, both adapted and pathological. This approach will be observed in terms of its therapeutic possibilities for the improvement and removal of the so-called negative symptoms. These are the warhorse for true recovery, understood as a personal and unique process for the clarification, development, adjustment of attitudes and values, affectivity and skills in social roles that can lead to a satisfactory and hopeful way of life. Those interventions that try to create a new existential situation or being-in-the-world will be described.

Keywords: Phenomenology, Psychosis, Schizophrenia, Values, Psychotherapy

1. Introduction

1.1 Theoretical foundation

Attempting to summarize the value structure in psychosis first requires defining three concepts: structure, values, and psychosis. Structure is understood as the relationship maintained between the different parts of a whole or the way in which said parts are organized in relation to the whole. For the purposes of the subject addressed in this work, the parts which we are concern with would be values. Their structure would determine the whole, which, as will be explained, is a reference to the *human person* [1, 2].

What are values? According to axiology—the philosophical discipline based on the value of things—values can be defined as those aspects that give meaning to things. Together, they will determine the behavior of an individual, depending on the importance they possess. Thus, values can be conceptualized as those attitudes whose function is to regulate our behavior. Surprisingly, however, despite being a key aspect in the construction of the individual, values have scarcely been studied in the field of psychosis [3].

The final element to define would be psychosis. The definition presented here will not address the well-known formal diagnostic systems (DSM-5 and ICD-11), albeit they are also classically discussed [4]. Instead, following a more phenomenological description, psychosis is understood more as a peculiar construction of the being-in-the-world, whose essential manifestation would be the "loss of common sense" or of natural evidence, caused by, among other factors, focusing on psychological processes that go unnoticed in other people [5, 6].

In this sense, it is also worth considering that the positive symptoms in psychosis (e.g., hallucinations, delusions, grossly disorganized or catatonic behavior) could well be the manifestation of more basic characteristics related to negative symptoms. Apathy, abulia and demotivation could in turn be the result of the lack of anchoring and fitting in with to the interests or social values of other people. In fact, it could be said that these negative symptoms are not simply located in the realm of affectivity; instead, they would exist as result of the specific relationship that the individual maintains with the oneself and towards the world. Both are not given separately or added but are to be understood as the basic being-in-the-world.

From this perspective, psychosis would be understood as the result of structural modifications of the self in its anchoring in the world-of-life, given the flaw in the construction of intersubjectivity and therefore common sense, understood as the basic intuitive tuning with the social world [6, 7].

1.2 Therapeutic approaches

In fact, the therapy session itself, not focused on the symptom, is the context that would present an opportunity for the development of intersubjectivity. The patient would have the chance to learn to feel what it is like to have things in common with others and experience feelings of acceptance and everyday life. Not in vain, the self-in-company is the barometer of the being-in-the-world [5].

In this regard, it is noteworthy that in recent years a great deal of therapeutic efforts made among patients with psychosis and severe mental disorders have resulted in strategies aimed precisely at attempting to restructure life's sense and, therefore, values. This approach leads to a more fulfilled life experience. For example, in the approach known as Open Dialog [8], listening emerges as a more important variable than the intervention method; it specifically allows the reduction of uncertainty while also revaluating the social support system. This grants greater responsibility to both the family and the patient to discuss life situations and to manage their lives more confidently.

Similarly, another alternative with phenomenological roots, practiced by mental health patients on their own, is the Power Threat Meaning Framework [9], a psychiatric diagnosis process proposed by the Division of Clinical Psychology of the British Psychological Society. In this case, symptoms would be understood as survival strategies against adversities and their meaning would always be related to life circumstances. Faced with threats (in relationships, identity, values, discrimination, emotions) generated by negative impacts of power (biological, coercive, legal, economic, cultural, interpersonal, or ideological forces), the patient will attempt to assign them meaning (beliefs, feelings, and physical reactions) and respond to them. These responses may include aggressive behavior, unusual sensory perceptual or cognitive experiences, catatonia, dissociation, hearing voices, weakness, affective flattening, indifference, submission, paranoia, panic, depersonalization or derealization, among others. The aim of this framework is to gather strength, enhance the socio/family support resources of each patient, in order to empower them and rebalance their life according to the values of justice, equity, personal safety, belonging, direction and agency. In this way, this approach would help patients to have an existence with sense, meaning and purpose. The above examples involve the generation of contexts that can revaluate existence, beyond traditional bio-medical framework.

In addition, it can also be proposed that delusions, alterations in discourse, the experience of corporeality and the temporality, paranoidal or schizoidal ways of interacting would be —once the phase of confusion had been overcome—completely self-evident to the psychotic person. This would be their personal "anchoring in the life-world". The need to anchor oneself —to be anchored—would imply that these phenomena would be evident to those individuals who lack common sense or the sense of belonging to the world of others. In fact, the *human person* model by [1] emphasizes the idea that the psychotic experience is a prototypically universal effort to construct a valuable and authentic sense of the self.

1.3 Life experiences of psychotic patients

However, any specific characteristics would stem from the complex experiences of the psychotic self which distance it precisely from certain socially adaptive values. They would therefore become barriers against achieving an acceptable level of wellbeing. Aspects related to work, sentimental relationships, raising a family, academic development and economic autonomy, leisure and social activities, health and general wellbeing tend to be either extraordinarily deficient or simply inexistent. It seems quite logical then that severe cases of psychosis appear during adolescence, precisely at a critical moment in the construction of the self. This development of the self would thus take place in the turbulent waters of the different conflictive roles (even ambivalent and antagonistic) which the individual will face as they evolve as a *person* [2].

Late-life psychosis also tends to develop in conflictive contexts or in complex existential transits, which would require a personal transformation not exempt from difficulties and risks. The Heideggerian concept of the human being as a transient and rational being and, therefore, narrative would imply the idea that living is always difficult. Overvaluation of the inner experience would result in an ontological catastrophe [10]. This private experience is a continuous flow of events, in which the event ("what *arrives*") impedes any feeling of having completely experienced what occurred [11]. This prompts the individual to experience events as not their own (since they are not *possessed*, and instead simply *appear*). Such events tend to be the object of overvaluation or hyper-reflexibility, whereby psychotic self-reflection is the "active stinger of the soul" [12]. In addition, this hyper-reflexibility occurs in different psychopathological conditions [13].

The life experience of certain psychotic individuals would therefore not cease to be a continuous and complex component. And that idiosyncratic environmental and behavioral history is what influences the experience of remembering, thinking, or feeling in the present. This refers to the world in which people exist; this world would arrive before the ideas created about it. This implies, in the words of Heidegger, that the individual must first remain "under the empire of Others".

The predefined types/models of life or values can be achieved, lived, understood, or accepted or not. It must be noted that values, as the guiding horizon which human beings migrate towards, and are therefore ingrained in them as psychological beings, cannot be reduced to a process of reasoning. Values cannot be accessed analytically because they *are there* (whether we want them or not). Thus, it is deduced that values will naturally be conditioned by different social-relational aspects.

1.4 Values of psychotic patients

It is important to consider some of the values engrained in the world of a person with psychosis when analyzing values. As previously discussed, their world is phenomenologically different from the common-sense world. It is normally associated with a sense of eccentricity or exceptional nature, which are believed to be "given", not chosen. In fact, it is observed that the axiological structure in psychosis features a preeminence of eschatological values that give great meaning to the life experience of patients. Thus, the feeling of idionomia or exceptionality and radical uniqueness is quite common [3]; the psychotic individual gives a meaning to events upon which they build a special –exceptional— identity. The events regulate their consciousness and life action, orienting them towards metaphysical existential planes, perhaps with a different mission or purpose from the objectives or goals common to their social environment. In Jaspers words [12] "the patient is personally important as a discoverer ... his days are filled with meaningful mental work". These eschatological values will be the center of gravity upon which the psychotic individual will sustain their actions and consciousness. This will remove them from other constitutive values which will probably remain frozen due to the enormity of their psychotic experience.

This disconnection from the pragmatic life and the distancing from the social-family context prevent the psychotic individual from learning essential lessons for interacting with the world. This peculiar case of self-absorption is common in modern societies [14]. According to Taylor [15], the dissolution of moral horizons, as a paradigm of modern society, would leave life with no ground to anchor itself onto given the loss of the sense provided by said horizons. In this way life could become what Nietzsche would called "a pitiful comfort" [15].

For example, a value that is usually common in a person with schizophrenia is spirituality. Their urgency to show it to others is common, so it is shared with everyone. As the objective of proselytism is to be praiseworthy a priori, it can also be characterized by a lack of empathic intuition; possibly generating a history of social rejection. These idiosyncratic values should not be easily confused with abnormal beliefs. Instead, they must be recognized as the world of the person in order to be modulated or adjusted in therapy [16]. This adjustment process would help the patient to untangle themselves from this egoic existential position. In turn, self-reflexivity would partially cease, allowing them to go beyond the oneself. This would result in an axiological reconstruction of the self by the *Self-for-Others*. The goal is not to invalidate the spiritual proselytism position, which is legitimate (we must remember that eschatological missions are not chosen *sensu stricto*, but are experienced as given), but rather to learn to experience sharing life, with no other function than to being-in-the world.

1.5 What patients suffer from

A common observation in the literature on the social integration of individuals with acute psychosis is the existence of severe problems with socio-labor insertion, intimacy, interpersonal communication, and sexuality. This results in a high level of suffering, which is substantially reduced when changes take place in these aspects [17]. The issue is that the lack of social experiences (from avoiding rejection, stigma, being misunderstood, etc.) impedes learning; it also complicates personal orientation towards other personal values. These are precisely the values which could be addressed at certain moments of the therapeutic process.

Survival against stigma, exclusion, and failure, due to the limitations that patients with psychosis suffer from, is a very complex situation. Competing within social function frameworks characterized by the paradigms of individualism and competitiveness is a serious problem, whereby achieving a valuable identity is a very difficult accomplishment. Therefore, it is quite likely to experience feelings of failure, inadequacy, shame, and exclusion, which are indeed forms of personal suffering [9].

Axiological structure will always involve a relationship of the world of the person with others. It involves social values that do not depend merely on individual decisions or processes; they are as much a part of the individual's difficulties and interests as the actual characteristics of their world. It must be noted that the world is lived on occasions as a whole, making it important to reconstruct the "real" or objective world, which would include friends (probably limited in number), family (generally highly conflictive) and the general population (with high levels of stigma, social distancing and rejection). We must bear in mind that the clarification of the value system is not an analytical dissection.

The "existential ground" where the ethical-moral structure is generated is not a series of items or reasons [15]. It is evident that this structure can and must be chosen, fully committing to the direction that each human being must take in their life. However, it should be noted that axiological structure is already given to us in the world we exist in. Thus, this existential structure of the *world-out-there* should also be clarified and wholeheartedly accepted.

It is also important to bear in mind that certain values could be conflictive in personal development. Some components of modern culture, whose maxim is self-realization and therefore emphasizes being "true to oneself", could specifically reinforce individualism and solipsist thinking. But this occurs not only in psychosis; eating disorders are an example of characterological formation based on perfectionism, control, and excessive individuation. Loyalty to that structure of egoic values, which can be useful on occasions, certainly limits and stifles existence itself [18]. Life could become clogged by a blindness to be "someone exceptional" (It will be pointed out, therefore, that any therapeutic effort should be directed to achieve a certain psychological flexibility that allows relativizing loyalty to this private world, above all if that position, both stubborn and defensive, distances the patient from the ordinary world of life).

2. Working with the axiological structure

2.1 Therapeutic dialog

In phenomenological approaches, it is understood that therapeutic sessions need not merely involve a logging of symptoms. Even initial phases, more focused on evaluation and establishing connection, are potentially valuable and enlightening moments. They can be used as opportunities to search for meaning and recognition – key moments for understanding and clarifying the value structure – from which a great deal a person's experience and actions originate [16].

As previously discussed, the therapeutic relationship itself is a magnificent opportunity to create a meaningful relationship. Even when listening and dialog first begins, contributions can be made towards developing a more robust, pre-reflexive self-awareness [19]. More than being in the presence of the contents of consciousness, it is a form of being that *comes before* them. To achieve greater existential adjustment, a dialogical transformation must occur as living is tantamount to being-in-the-world. Intersubjectivity is enhanced during the process of mutual recognition, which is such a convulsive aspect of the psychotic experience. In this way, the value structure that moves the person can be understood, making it possible to equip patients with greater psychological flexibility. This will be necessary to both identify values and reveal the common conflicts between them.

The key is, if axiological structure regulates behavior, then its adjustment will allow greater empowerment for a better existential commitment. The literature establishes that psychological recovery among this population refers to establishing commitments, which must focus on constructing a life with meaning, as well as a positive sense of identity. According to [20], the experience of oneself must be based on hope and self-determination. The therapeutic process encourages hope, redefines the identity based on an existential sense and helps the patient to take responsibility for their recovery. This must be approached as an ethical-moral orientation, that is, as a philosophy or life orientation [21]. Therapeutic progress is more than the reduction of positive symptoms; it is a way of being in front them, in front oneself and in front of the world-of-life.

2.2 Clarification of values

However, this world is difficult though because, as Jaspers states, living is a "controversy with the world". There is always difficulty when reorganizing the value structure, whether addressing the level of confusion, disinformation, or disorganization that the psychotic individual has over themselves. Yet, it is important to highlight one of the key life experiences in the existence of a person with psychosis: fear and suffering, in either the present (oppression, anguish, confusion, stigma) or co-present (avoidance of intimacy, apathy, laughter out of context, metaphysical stubbornness, distancing from the world).

An additional difficulty in the value identification process tends to be the defensive disguising of intense malaise. That co-present fear, hidden or even buried in cognitive-emotional paralysis or in one's own self-absorption, needs to be lived and made conscious so it may be elaborated, understood, and accepted. This is a basic therapeutic condition that makes it possible to advance beyond the unrevealing of personal values.

Even apathy could be understood as a way of being. The function of this way of being-in-the-world would provide a sort of anesthesia for feeling. When a feeling is incomprehensible, unmanageable, or experienced with strangeness, it is to be expected that they will flee from it. The proposal would be to face these phenomena of living; everything has a purpose, meaning and function. The conflicts derived from the experience of fear allow more effective access to the world of values and their personal worth [9].

If the experience of constructing a sense of the self is eminently intersubjective, it is necessary to create non-invalidating meeting spaces, both in the therapeutic setting and in the formation of natural groups. Experiencing identity includes an axiological structure that must be identified to produce a practical self-knowledge that allows the patient to know how to direct their own life. In this sense, it is worth noting that discussion about the meaning of values benefits from a natural framework, featuring, for example, the participation of more therapists, mutual support groups and family, as in the *Open Dialogue* approach [8].

Giving the patient with responsibility implies respect for their opinions and their participation throughout the entire process. There is evidence of a therapeutic benefit showing that clinics help to generate different perspectives in which these values in conflict can coexist [22].

2.3 Values and therapy

Thus, therapeutic approaches that could offer an opportunity to identify axiological structure in this population, observe conflicts between the values at play and empower the psychotic patient to deal with obstacles in order to have a life committed to said values, would be those which:

- Seek to capture subjective aspects, namely, the phenomenological experience of the person, removed from psychopathological categories.

- Observe the complexity of life itself and explore feelings, values, personal meaning and experience.

- Accompany the patient in the difficult commitment of choosing their life, accepting the unfinished aspects of their life project.

- Disentangle from their mental processes when self-reflexivity fails to help them transcend.

- Allow ambiguity, as this will teach the patient to tolerate it.

- Successfully manage to make therapeutic contact truly meaningful, creating a comprehensive space that allows patients to feel and do from within themselves; therapist and patient can always present interpretations from the *being-in-the-world* of the patient (their self and the particular circumstances).

- Allow the patient to experience desperation, in order to understand their stagnation and the feeling of blocking or impairment of the horizon of their future; only from there can the patient collaborate in their own activation towards life, when that is precisely their goal.

- Follow the idiosyncratic scripts of life and that which occurs in therapeutic here-now relationships, rather than prejudicial constructs.

The therapist will be an example of Other in the relationship history of the patient; this will be crucial to the change process given the importance of Others in the construction of the person, as previously explained. For this reason, it will be necessary to address the basic components of the therapeutic session: material production (essentially verbal behavior, but other types of interpersonal behaviors as well, of course), analysis (essentially comprehensive) and the therapeutic relationship (alliance and closeness).

All resistance will be understood as kinds of behavior which make attempts at experiential avoidance. It will be necessary to understand and respect them so they can be addressed when the psychotic individual is ready. In this way will be reminded that these behaviors function as protective strategies that have been assigned meaning.

The change in therapy should not be directed to stop being who one is, but to live with another perspective in the face of the challenges of one's own existence. Some of these challenges are the construction of a valuable identity and the search for meaning of what happens. And this will always be done on the fundamental basis of the person: the axiological structure of him.

3. Conclusion

The phenomenological perspective on how to understand psychotic problems makes it possible to stay ahead of phenomena precisely as they occur. Doing so avoids prejudiced constructs that obscure the *there-given* [23]. It eliminates representational aporias and mechanistic paradigm removing them from the experiences of patients with psychosis. In this way, models focused on the *human person* [1, 2] understand psychotic experiences as phenomena linked to normal psychological development.

People with psychosis will make a great effort to construct a valuable sense of themselves. They understand themselves according to their life experience, in which they construct their social identity and their self in a context; this is the being-in-the-world.

While making this effort, their behavior would deviate from practical actions in life, receiving responses of rejection, stigma, and failure, keeping them even further distanced and absorbed in their private events. Their axiological structure would remain in a state of adolescence or frozen.

The therapy process could help to clarify and endow the patient with more adaptive personal values. It is necessary to provide and find therapeutic settings that allow the meaningful experience of identity to be valuable, reconnecting the patient with the *world-there-given* as a horizon. It is important to make the transition from the prototypical monological life experience of schizophrenia to a dialogical one. The phenomenological approach is undoubtedly one of the most encouraging comprehension and intervention perspectives for this type of mental health problems. It is responsible for verifying that the recovery of negative and emotional symptoms, as well as the emotional component of psychotic experiences, are related to socio-community functioning and obtaining a valuable life experience [24].

The phenomenological perspective would also be at the base of the new movements in mental health. *The Open Dialogue* or Hearing Voices approaches emphasize the experience of the person and the problematic experiences. They allow to understand them in the social and family context. The processes of psychological change are related to present values.

Likewise, in phenomenological approaches the value of the symptoms is inserted in the life of the person. For this reason, the work on negative symptoms, basic in the axiological anchoring of the person, becomes highly relevant.

Author details

Francisco Martín-Murcia* and Adolfo J. Cangas
University of Almería, Almería, Spain

*Address all correspondence to: psicologo@me.com

References

[1] Chadwick P, Birchow M, Trower P (1996). Cognitive therapy for ilusions, voices and paranoia. Chichester: Wiley. 346 p. 1996.

[2] García-Montes. JM, Pérez-Álvarez M. Reivindicación de la persona en la esquizofrenia (Claiming the person in schizophrenia). International Journal of Clinical and Health Psychology. 2002; 3: 107-122.

[3] Stanghellini G, Ballerini M. Values in persons with schizophrenia. Schizophrenia Bulletin. 2007; 33:131-141. DOI: org/10.1093/schbul/sbl036. DOI: 10.1093/oxforddhb/97801988031 57.001.0001.

[4] Boyle M. The Non-Discovery of Schizophrenia. Kraepelin and Bleuler reconsidered. In: R.P. Bentall RP, editor. Reconstructing Schizophrenia. London: Routledge. 1990. p. 3-22.

[5] Blankenburg W. La pérdida de la evidencia natural: una contribución a la psicopatología de la esquizofrenia (The loss of natural evidence: a contribution to the psychopathology of schizophrenia). Santiago de Chile: Ediciones Universidad Diego. 2013.

[6] Stanghellini G. Disembodied spirit and deanimated bodies. Oxford, UK: Oxford University Press. 2006. 225 p. DOI: 10.1093/med/9780198520894.001.0001.

[7] Nelson B, Sass LA, Thompson A, Yung AR, Francey SM, Amminger GP, McGorry PD. Does disturbance of self underlie social cognition deficits in schizophrenia and other psychotic disorders? Early Intervention in Psychiatry. 2009; 3:83-93. DOI: 10.111/j.1751-7893.2009.00112.x.

[8] Galbusera L, Kyselo M. The difference that makes the difference: a conceptual analysis of the open dialogue approach. Psychosis. 2018; 10: 47-54. DOI:org/10.1080/17522439.2017.1397734.

[9] Johnstone L, Boyle M, Cromby J, Dillon J, Harper D, Kinderman P, Longden E, Pilgrim D, Read J. The Power Threat Meaning Framework: Overview. Leicester: British Psychological Society. 2018.414 p.

[10] Dastur F. La ipseidad: su importancia en la psicopatología (Ipseity: its importance to psychopatology). Universitas Philosophica. 2015; 32:251-266. DOI: 10.11144/Javeriana.uph32-64.iipp.

[11] Rovaletti ML (2014). Psicopatología Fenomenológica Contemporánea (Contemporary Phenomenological Psychopathology). VI Congreso Internacional de Psicopatología Fundamental e XII Congresso Brasileiro de Psicopatología Fundamental and Associaciao Universitaria de Pesquisa em Psicopatología Fundamental. 4-7 September 2014; Belo Horizonte, Brasil.

[12] Jaspers K. Psicopatología General (General Psychopathology). México: Fondo de Cultura Económica. 1993. 962 p.

[13] Pérez-Álvarez M. Hyperreflexivity as condition in mental disorders: A clinical and historical perspective. Psicothema. 2008; 20: 181-187.

[14] Sass LA. Madness and modernism. Insanity in the light of modern art, literature, and thought. Cambridge: Harvard University Press. 1992. 595 p.

[15] Taylor C. The ethics of authenticity. Cambridge, Mass: Harvard University Press. 1991. 4-160 p.

[16] Mancini M, Stanghellini G. Values in persons with bordeline personality disorder: their relevance for the therapeutic interview. Research in

Pychoterapy: Psychopatology, Process and Outcome. 2020; 23: 48-55. DOI: org/10.4081/ripppo.2020.449.

[17] Sahu KK. Intervening Negative Impact of Stigma on Employability of a Person with Schizophrenia Through Social Case Work. Journal of Psychosocial Rehabilitation and Mental Health, 2015; 2: 87-95. DOI: 10.1007/s40737-015-0029-2.

[18] Bloom A. The Closing of the American Mind. New York: Simon & Schuster. 1988. 400 p.

[19] García Montes JM, Pérez-Álvarez M, Sass L. La hora de la fenomenología en la esquizofrenia (The time of phenomenology in schizophrenia). Clínica y Salud. 2010; 21: 221-233. DOI: 10.5093/cl2010v21n3a2.

[20] Andresen R, Oades L, Caputi P. The experience of recovery from schizophrenia: towards an empirical validated state model. Australian and New Zealand Journal of Psychiatry. 2003; 37:586-594. DOI: 10.1046/j.1440-1614.2003.01234.x

[21] Leamy M, Bird V, Le Boutillier C, Willians J, Slade, N. Conceptual framework for personal recovery in mental health: Systematic review and narrative synthesis. British Journal of Psychiatry. 2011;199: 445-452. DOI: 10.1192/bjp.bp.110.083733.

[22] Stanghellini G, Broome M, Fernández AV, Fusar-Poli P, Raballo A, Rosfort R. (2019). The Oxford Handbook of Phenomenological Psychopathology. New York: Oxford University Press and Guilford Press. 2019. 1184 p. DOI: 10.1093/oxforddhb/9780198803157.001.0001.

[23] Martín-Murcia F, Ferro, R. Phenomenology and Psychopatology in Third Generation Therapies. Psychology, Society, & Education. 2015; 7, 97-106. DOI: 10.25115/psye.v7i1.543.

[24] Best M, Law H, Pyle M, Morrison A. Relationships between psychiatric symptoms, functioning and personal recovery in psychosis. Schizophrenia Research. 2020; 223:112-118. DOI: 10.1016/j.schres.2020.0626.

Section 2

Psychopathology

Chapter 3

Clinical Staging in Schizophrenia Spectrum Disorders

Zsófia Borbála Dombi, Ágota Barabássy, Barbara Sebe, István Laszlovszky and György Németh

Abstract

The aim of this chapter is to summarize the state-of-the-art knowledge of clinical staging in schizophrenia spectrum disorders. Clinical staging has been introduced to psychiatry in the past two decades. Its primary goal is to divide the course of the disorder into recognizable stages based on seriousness, development and symptom characteristics in order to better predict prognosis and to adopt the most appropriate treatment strategies. The first staging model was developed in 1982. Since then several distinct concepts of clinical staging in psychiatry have emerged. To date, there is no clinical consensus regarding which staging model is the gold standard, nonetheless when merging them together an integrated staging concept arises. The integrated staging model of schizophrenia spectrum disorders is composed of four stages. The chapter will introduce the different staging models in a historical order as well as present the integrated staging model detailing the characteristics, timeline and dominating symptoms of each stage. Appropriate treatment strategies for the distinct stages will also be outlined.

Keywords: schizophrenia spectrum disorders, clinical staging

1. Introduction

Schizophrenia spectrum disorders (SSD) are a collection of psychotic disorders defined by abnormalities in one or more of the following symptom domains: hallucinations, delusions, disorganized thinking, catatonic behavior and negative symptoms [1]. The word 'spectrum' has been first added in the fifth edition of the Diagnostic and Statistical Manual of Mental Disorders (DSM-V) [1, 2], reflecting the notion that psychiatric disorders lie on a spectrum with no sharp boundaries between them [3, 4]. According to the DSM-V, SSD include schizophrenia, schizophreniform disorder, schizoaffective disorder, delusional disorder, brief psychotic disorder, psychotic disorders due to another medical condition or substance/medication, and unspecified or specified schizophrenia spectrum and other psychotic disorders [1]. The prevalence rate for SSD is estimated to be 7 per 1000 [5], with higher rates in men than in women [6]. Currently, there are over 21 million people who are affected by this condition [7]. Diagnosis is made along a spectrum of symptoms and severity via clinical interviews as no confirmatory and diagnostic laboratory nor radiological tests are available [2]. Although schizophrenia represents only about one third of the SSD cases [8], it is the most researched disorder out of all [9].

Besides the internationally used diagnostic systems such as DSM or the International Classification of Diseases (ICD), there is another, complementary form of classifying psychiatric disorders called clinical staging [10]. First introduced in cardiology and oncology [11], clinical staging is different from the conventional diagnostic practices in a sense that it does not only define the extent of illness progression but also where a patient lies within the course of the disorder [10]. The basic assumptions of clinical staging are that (a) treatment in the early stages of the disorder is more efficient, (b) patients experience greater symptom severity in the later stages of the illness, and (c) the process of transferring to a later stage is connected with a typical clinical profile [12]. Although clinical staging as a model for classifying the development of disorders had been ignored in psychiatry in the past, several concepts have emerged in the past few decades [11]. The primary aim of clinical staging is promoting recovery in the early stages of psychiatric disorders as well as preventing progression to later stages [10]. Importantly, clinical stages of psychiatric disorders can be defined by many different aspects from symptom severity and persistence, through neurobiological changes, to the emotional processes that happen within the patient [10]. In this chapter, we aim to present, summarize and synthetize the clinical staging concepts of SSD through a systematic review.

2. Clinical staging concepts of schizophrenia spectrum disorders

The systematic review was conducted in November 2020 using the MEDLINE, EMBASE and Cochrane databases from 1999 with the following search terms: 'stage/staging', combined using the Boolean 'AND' operator with 'psychiatric disorder/schizophrenia/ psychosis/psychotic disorder'. Additionally, a manual search was also performed. Titles and abstracts were screened by one of the authors (Zs.D.) and relevant articles were independently assessed by two authors (A.B. and Zs.D.). English-language articles published in peer-reviewed journals describing complete staging models on SSD or psychiatric disorders, in general, were eligible to be included in the chapter (inclusion critera).

As a result of the systematic search, a total of 2045 articles were identified. After reviewing the abstracts to exclude those which clearly did not meet the above-mentioned criteria, 27 articles remained. Of these, 9 articles were included in the final review.

2.1 The Hoffman staging concept

Although most reviews do not count the staging model of schizophrenia proposed by Brian Hoffman in 1982, it can be considered to be the first attempt to divide the course of the disorder into recognizable stages [11, 13]. In his concept, Hoffman described the stages of schizophrenia based on the patient's reaction to his or her symptoms, beginning with anxiety (stage 1) and ending with acceptance (stage 5) (**Figure 1**) [13]. In the early phase of schizophrenia, before the first episode, the patient goes through considerable changes in their behavior and experience disturbance in thinking which can result in fear and anxiety or even anger [13]. Then, during the first episode of schizophrenia, the patient experiences a stage of denial (stage 2) where they no longer acknowledge that they have problem mainly due to excessive positive symptoms [13]. The third stage is about ambivalence, where the patients begin to have some insight into their disorder but might reject medication and go through multiple hospitalizations [13]. Before the final stage, acceptance (stage 5), there is a stage of depression (stage 4) where the

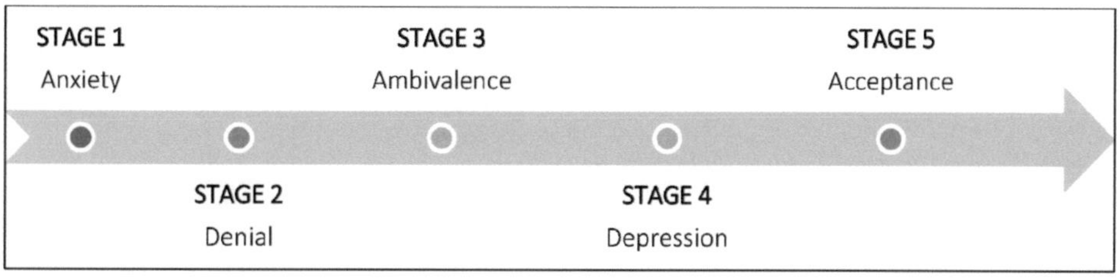

Figure 1.
The Hoffman staging concept.

patient realizes the seriousness of the disorder [13]. During this stage it is important to monitor the patient to prevent suicide and alter the medication doses accordingly [13]. Although this staging concept is different from the others, it recognizes the importance of taking into account the patient's emotional response to his or her symptoms and the progression of the disorder which is now considered vital in a modern, person-centered care [14].

2.2 The Fava and Kellner staging concept

The first staging model of schizophrenia is attributed to Fava and Kellner who proposed their concept in 1993 [11, 15]. According to their model, schizophrenia starts with a prodromal stage (stage 1), where mainly negative and affective symptoms are present with considerable deterioration in functioning (**Figure 2**) [15]. The second stage is the acute episode of schizophrenia, dominated by positive symptoms [15]. The residual or third stage is described by the absence of positive symptoms and increased presentation of negative symptoms (resembling to stage 1) [15]. Finally, the authors differentiate between subchronic (stage 4) and chronic (stage 5) phases based on the duration of the illness; if it persists more than 6 months but less than 2 years then it is stage 4, if it is present for more than 2 years then it is stage 5 [15]. Additionally, it is also emphasized that a "rollback phenomenon" can also occur where patients in stage 2 progress to stage 1 instead of stage 3 and achieve remission eventually [15].

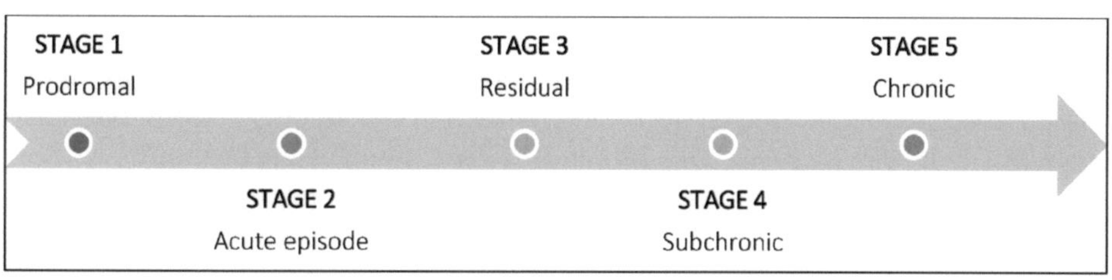

Figure 2.
The Fava & Kellner staging concept.

2.3 The staging concepts of Lieberman and Insel

According to Lieberman, schizophrenia is composed of three pathophysiologic phases described in four stages [11, 16]. The first is the neurodevelopmental or premorbid phase which begins in early adolescence or even sooner and is characterized by mild cognitive and social impairments (stage 1) (**Figure 3**) [16]. Then the second phase is the neuroplastic phase which can be further divided into prodromal, and onset and deterioration sub-phases and is referred to as stage 2 and 3 in the model,

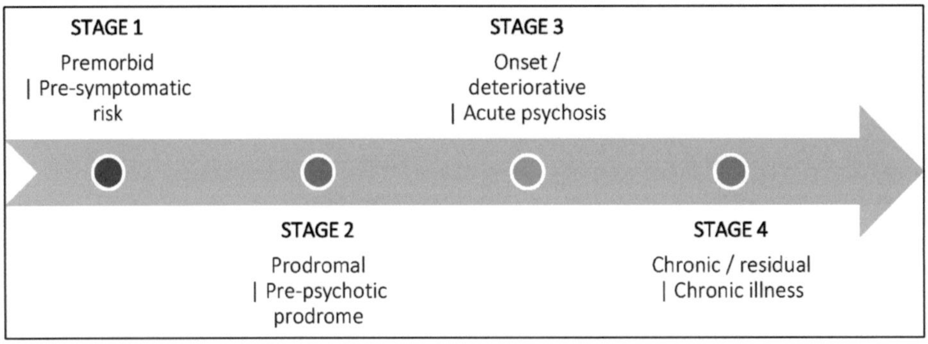

Figure 3.
The staging concepts of Lieberman and Insel.

accordingly [16]. Throughout the prodromal stage besides the above mentioned deficits, mild psychotic symptoms might be already present which lead to a full-blown psychosis during the onset (stage 3) [16]. The final pathophysiological phase is the neuroprogressive one, which is described as the chronic or residual stage characterized by considerable negative and cognitive symptoms as well as further psychotic episodes [16]. Lieberman recommends the use of antipsychotic medication only after the onset of the first psychotic episode [16]. Similarly, to Lieberman, 9 years later Insel also identified the same stages of schizophrenia albeit with slightly different names; pre-symptomatic risk (stage 1), pre-psychotic prodrome (stage 2), acute psychosis (stage 3) and chronic illness (stage 4) [17, 18]. In his staging concept, he also details the features, diagnosis, disability and intervention at each distinct stage [17].

2.4 The Singh staging concept

The staging concept by Singh and colleagues focuses predominantly on the chronology of psychosis onset [19]. Their model beings with the prodrome (stage 1), which is further divided into two parts; a period of unease (P1) and a period of non-diagnostic symptoms (P2) [19]. Then, the second stage is when the first psychotic symptoms appear, which refers to positive symptoms such as delusions and hallucinations [19]. Before receiving a definite diagnosis (stage 4), there is an intermediate stage where the symptoms build up, and there is already a diagnostic impression of schizophrenia (stage 3) [19]. Although this staging concept does not describe a complete model of SSD, its detailed description of the beginning of the disorder made it worthy of being included in this review (**Figure 4**).

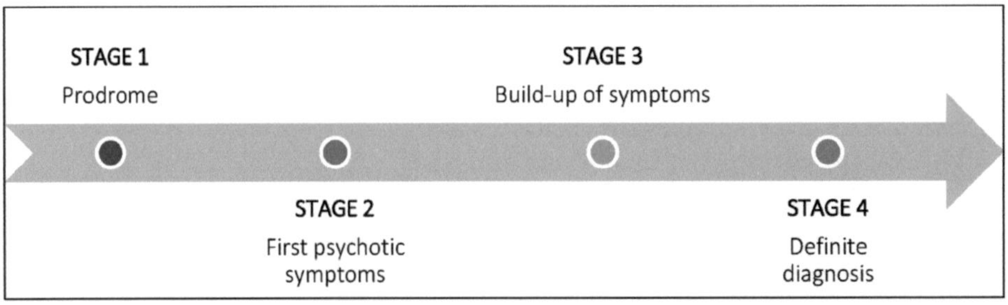

Figure 4.
The Singh staging concept.

2.5 The Agius staging concept

The simplest and probably most known concept of schizophrenia staging was described by Agius after about a decade of the Lieberman model [12]. Based on his research, the development of schizophrenia was divided into three distinct stages; the prodrome (stage 1), then the first episode (stage 2) and finally, the chronic phase (stage 3) (**Figure 5**) [12]. Although it was not included in the model as a separate stage, Agius also agrees on the fact that there is a premorbid phase before the prodrome [12]. It is also emphasized that the treatment of schizophrenia needs to be in accordance with the different stages of the disorder in order to achieve the desired outcomes [12].

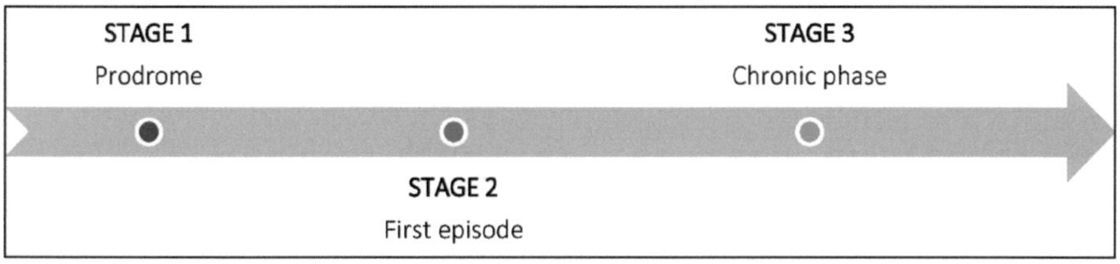

Figure 5.
The Agius staging concept.

2.6 The McGorry staging concept

One of the most developed and referenced [20–24] staging model of schizophrenia was proposed by McGorry and colleagues [10, 11]. This concept starts with stage 0, where the patient has no current symptoms yet, but an increased risk of psychotic disorder is present (**Figure 6**) [10]. Then, stage 1 (mild and moderate symptoms) is divided into two substages; 1a with mild and non-specific symptoms and 1b with subthreshold or moderate symptoms [10]. The first episode of psychosis defined to be at stage 2, followed by the three substages of stage 3 (incomplete remission and relapse(s)); incomplete remission (3a), relapse of psychotic disorder (3b) and multiple relapses (3c) [10]. Finally, stage 4 represents a persistent and severe illness [10]. Importantly, this staging concept can be applied not only to patients with SSD but also to patients with other severe mood disorders such as depression or bipolar disorder [10]. Besides the description of different stages, McGorry and colleagues also provided information regarding the potential interventions as well as indicative biological and endophenotypic markers to each stage in their framework [10].

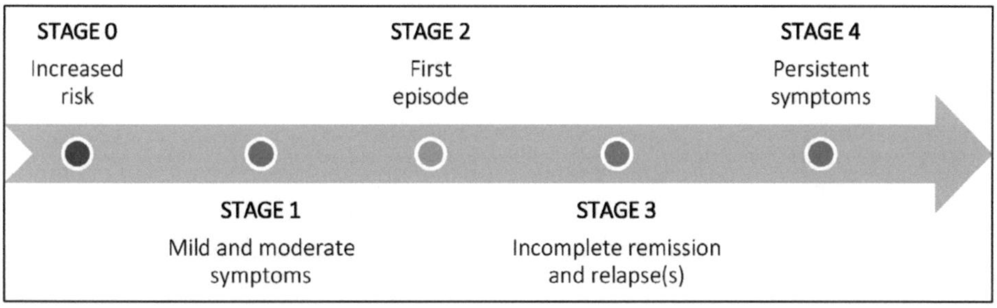

Figure 6.
The McGorry staging concept.

2.7 The Cosci staging concept

In 2013, Cosci and colleagues – similarly to this book chapter – aimed to summarize and integrate the staging models of schizophrenia, and other major psychiatric disorders through a systematic review and came up with a general staging concept that is composed of four stages (**Figure 7**) [11]. The model starts with a prodromal phase (stage 1) and follows the basic stages of psychiatric disorders in a longitudinal fashion with stage 2 being the acute manifestation, stage 3 the residual phase and stage 4 the chronic phase [11]. In contrast to McGorry [10] and Lieberman [16], the premorbid or increased risk phase was not included in this concept as they found no adequate support from the literature and argued that it has less clinical relevance as it can be only appraised retrospectively [11].

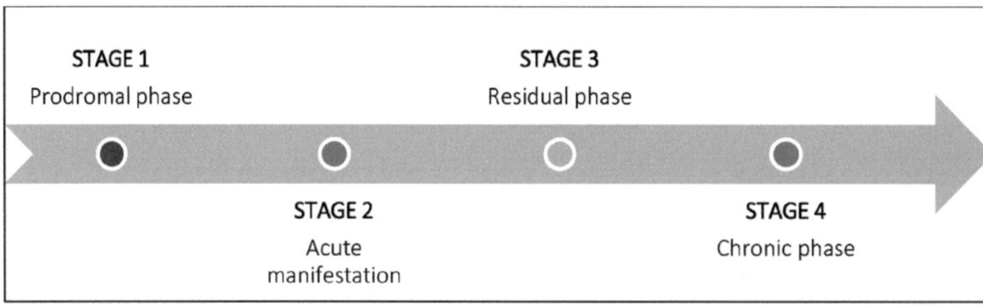

Figure 7.
The Cosci staging concept.

2.8 The Fountoulakis staging concept

A novel concept of clinical staging in schizophrenia was proposed by Fountoulakis and colleagues in 2019 using the Positive and Negative Syndrome Scale (PANSS) and the 5-factor model (a model based on the notion that schizophrenia is characterized by positive, negative, cognitive, affective and hostility symptoms) [25]. They aimed to develop a staging concept empirically through analyzing a very large sample (n = 2358) of stabilized schizophrenia patients with varying ages [25]. Based on the results, they identified 4 major stages of schizophrenia (**Figure 8**), starting with stage 1, dominated by positive symptoms. Besides describing the most influential symptom domain of each stage, they also provided a timeline of the disorder. According to this timeline, stage 1 lasts about 3 years on average [25]. In this first stage, excitement and hostility symptoms were found to increase over time and becoming the leading symptom group of stage 2, that lasts

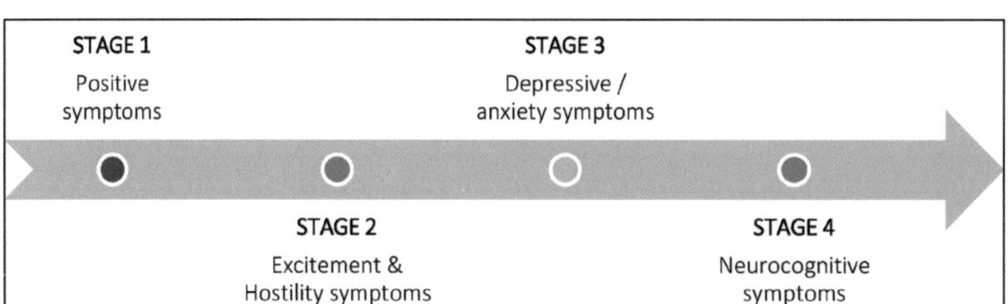

Figure 8.
The Fountoulakis staging concept.

about 9 years on average [25]. Throughout the first two stages, negative and depression/ anxiety symptoms were stable and started to increase steadily around the end of stage 2 [25]. Importantly, the second stage was further divided into 2 substages: stage 2a and 2b [25]. The latter lasts about 6 years and is described by the rise of negative, depressive and cognitive symptoms. During stage 3, which lasted 13 years on average, the most dominant symptoms were the depressive ones [25]. In the first phase of stage 3 (3a), hostility symptoms were found to decline, while negative and cognitive symptoms were increasing [25]. Then, in the second part of stage 3 (3b), positive and hostility symptoms almost disappeared [25]. Finally, the fourth stage was found to be characterized by cognitive symptoms, and according to their timeline, it begins 25 years after the first episode on average [25]. Similarly to the previous stages, stage 4 is also divided into 4a and 4b substages; 4a lasts about 15 years on average and is described by the robust increase of negative and cognitive symptoms, while 4b starts about 40 years after the first onset and is found to be dominated by mainly the neurocognitive deficits that the patients experience [25].

2.9 Similarities and differences between the historical staging concepts

A summary of the reviewed historical staging models of SSD is presented in **Table 1**. Interestingly, only about half of the staging concepts begin with a premorbid phase (Singh starts with prodrome which has a sub-stage, P1, that can be regarded as a premorbid phase), and except Fountoulakis and colleagues, all models have a prodromal phase. Importantly, the acute and chronic phase is present in all models (the Singh staging concept is not counted here, as it focused on the beginning of the disorder), while only again about half of the models included a residual or subchronic phase. In terms of the underlying pathophysiological changes of SSD in relation to the different stages, evidence from brain imaging studies provide support for the general notion that abnormalities are more prevalent in later stages than in earlier ones, these abnormalities are progressively worsening while patients advance from an earlier to a later stage and finally, supportive treatments such as essential fatty acid supplementation are more effective in the beginning of the disorder [26, 27]. Nonetheless, it is challenging to validate one particular model via pathophysiological changes described by brain abnormalities or other biomarkers as there is considerable heterogeneity in the clinical and pathophysiological picture of SSDs [27]. For instance, the size of the ventricles does not necessarily correlate with the severity or progression of symptoms nor signposts the patient's response to treatment [27].

	Premorbid phase	**Prodromal phase**	**Acute phase**	**Residual phase**	**Chronic phase**
Hoffman	Stage 1	Stage 2	Stage 3	Stage 4	Stage 5
	Anxiety	Denial	Ambivalence	Depression	Acceptance
Fava & Kellner		Stage 1	Stage 2	Stage 3–4	Stage 5
		Prodromal	Acute episode	Residual & Subchronic	Chronic
Lieberman	Stage 1	Stage 2	Stage 3		Stage 4
	Premorbid	Prodromal	Onset / deteriorative		Chronic / residual
Insel	Stage 1	Stage 2	Stage 3		Stage 4
	Pre-symptomatic risk	Pre-psychotic prodrome	Acute psychosis		Chronic illness

	Premorbid phase	Prodromal phase	Acute phase	Residual phase	Chronic phase
Singh	Stage 1 (P1)	Stage 1 (P2)	Stage 2–4		
	Prodrome	Prodrome	First psychotic symptoms & Build-up of symptoms & Definite diagnosis		
Agius		Stage 1	Stage 2		Stage 3
		Prodrome	First episode		Chronic phase
McGorry	Stage 0	Stage 1	Stage 2	Stage 3	Stage 4
	Increased risk	Mild and moderate symptoms	First episode	Incomplete remission and relapse(s)	Persistent symptoms
Cosci		Stage 1	Stage 2	Stage 3	Stage 4
		Prodromal phase	Acute manifestation	Residual phase	Chronic phase
Fountoulakis			Stage 1–2	Stage 3	Stage 4
			Positive, excitement & hostility symptoms	Depressive & anxiety symptoms	Neuro-cognitive symptoms

Table 1.
Summary of the reviewed staging concepts.

3. The integrated staging model of schizophrenia spectrum disorders

Although the reviewed historical staging concepts of SSD are slightly different from one another, they can easily be integrated into one coherent model. To start with, there is one clinical stage that is present in all concepts: the first episode of psychosis. This acute phase can be interpreted as a milestone that divides the course of the disorder into a *before* and an *after* phase and so can be set as the first stage of the disorder. It is also the stage where the patient is most likely to be recognized and treated for the first time.

Most, but not all clinical staging concepts deal with the *before* phase, officially called the prodrome, since it is often determined retrospectively and is highly debated from the perspective of treatment [11]. Nonetheless, evidence is emerging regarding early interventions and it might become more and more relevant in the future [28]. Hence, in the integrated staging model, the prodromal phase is regarded as stage 0, representing its importance but debated nature. In many of the reviewed staging models, prodrome was further divided into substages, i.e. increased risk or pre-morbid phase, and mild symptoms or prodromal phase [10, 16, 17]. Although these substages might be important in the development of SSD, recognizing them may be even more challenging and unnaturalistic in real-life settings [11, 28, 29]. Thus, in the integrated model, this stage is not subdivided further.

Similarly, to the *before* phase, there are slight differences between the historical staging concepts in terms of what happens *after* the first onset of psychotic symptoms. Some argue that there is only one stage after the acute manifestation

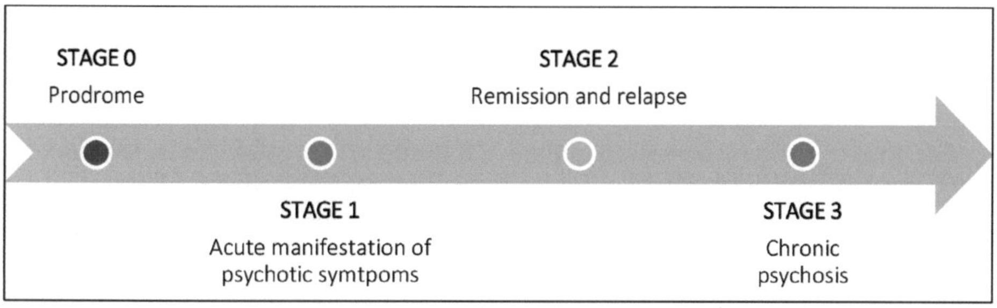

Figure 9.
The intergraded staging model of schizophrenia spectrum disorders.

of symptoms [12, 16, 17] while others define three or even more distinct stages [13, 15, 25]. The most influential models opt however for two subsequent stages [10, 11, 19]; a residual or pre-chronic stage characterized by incomplete remission, relapses as well as depressive symptoms, and a chronic stage with persistent symptoms dominated by neurocognitive deficits. In the integrated staging model these phases represent stage 2 (remission and relapse) and 3 (chronic psychosis), respectively (**Figure 9**).

3.1 The prodrome (stage 0)

In the integrated staging model of SSD, stage 0 is called the prodrome. This is a period of the disorder when some mild or even moderate symptoms are present, however there is no sign of full-blown psychosis yet [10]. Given the fact that this phase is just preceding the first onset of psychotic symptoms, the prodrome is a retrospective concept that can be mainly recognized and defined afterwards [28, 29]. In terms of timeline, the prodrome can last from weeks to even years, but most typically, its duration is about a year [28].

During the prodrome, the patient goes through considerable changes in their behavior and might start to experience disturbance in thinking which in turn results in anxiety or even anger [13]. The symptoms present during this time are heterogenous; mostly negative symptoms such as anhedonia, asociality or amotivation along with changes in perception, mood, beliefs and cognition [29, 30]. In terms of neurobiological changes, there are signs of abnormal dopamine synthesis, prefrontal cortex (PFC) dysfunctions and gray matter volume reductions in several brain regions including the PFC, hippocampal gyrus and lateral temporal lobe [31–34].

Given the notion that the earlier the treatment is received, the better the prognosis of SSD, there is considerable interest in starting pharmacological interventions during the prodrome [28, 29]. However, the main problem with this concept is the potential number of false positives, those individuals who, despite having symptoms and distress, will not develop psychosis after the prodromal period [29]. Thus, many argue that prescribing antipsychotic medication to these individuals is highly questionable from an ethical perspective, claiming that even the newest antipsychotic medications are not without side effects, might induce cognitive harm and can stigmatize the patient for life [28, 29, 35].

To overcome the barrier of treating individuals in the prodrome while also excluding the false positives, there are tendencies of developing new criteria that can accurately detect patients who are in an 'ultra-high risk' (UHR) mental state and hence are most likely to develop psychosis and benefit from pharmacological treatment too [29, 36]. An example of such criteria is the Personal Assessment and Crisis Evaluation (PACE), which defines someone at UHR of psychosis if they have one or more of the following diagnosis; "(a) attenuated psychotic symptoms, (b) brief limited intermittent psychotic symptoms, (c) a significant decrease in functioning (maintained for at least a month) with either schizotypal personality disorder or a first-degree relative with psychotic disorder" [28, 36, 37].

The aims of early intervention in the UHR group are threefold: first, to alleviate the symptoms that the patient experiences; second, to decrease the risk of transitioning to a first episode of psychosis; and third, to reduce the time before starting an antipsychotic treatment after the onset of psychosis [36]. To date, there are only a few pharmacological trials with antipsychotic medication in this patient group, both indicating a tendency for a decreased rate of conversion to psychosis after one year [38, 39]. Nonetheless, more research is required to understand the risks and benefits of pharmacological treatment during the UHR period. Meanwhile, according to current guidelines the use of antipsychotic medication during the prodrome is only recommended in case of the more complex cases [40, 41], while the recommended interventions are family psychoeducation, individual or group cognitive behavior therapy, active substance use reduction and neuroprotective agents such as omega-3 [10].

3.2 The onset (stage 1)

The first stage of the integrated staging model of SSD starts with the acute manifestation of psychotic symptoms or in other words the onset of the first episode of psychosis. Throughout this stage of the disorder patients experience predominantly positive symptoms such as hallucinations, paranoia or delusions and are likely to be in denial of accepting that there is something wrong and that they need medical help [10, 13]. This denial often manifests in aggression or agitation and might as well result in the hospitalization of the patient [42]. Besides the dominating positive symptoms, negative symptoms such as alogia or asociality and hostility may also be present [16, 25].

Currently, there is no strong scientific evidence on the cut-off point for the end of the first episode, nonetheless, it is estimated to be within the first 2–5 years following the onset of the psychotic symptoms [43–45]. Indeed, Fountoulakis and colleagues found that the first stage of SSD lasts 3 years on average [25].

The main treatment goal during the first stage of SSD is to resolve psychotic symptoms and to increase the chances of the patients to returning to their normal life as effectively and expeditiously as possible [41]. To do so, antipsychotic medications are utilized [46], in most cases in the form of oral antipsychotics due to being less invasive and more accepted in the long run [47]. Many patients, however, might need long-acting, injectable antipsychotics in order to increase compliance [48], as several studies indicated that more than 40% of patients are nonadherent during the first 9 months of treatment, hence increasing their chance to relapse [49].

In addition to pharmacological treatment it is also important to provide further support to the patients and their caregivers via clinical psychologists, occupational therapists and social workers [10, 41]. The family or caregivers might need to attend psychoeducation or other therapy as well in order to ensure better coping [41].

After the first episode, there are multiple trajectories possible how the disorder can continue. According to the thumb rule described by Shepherd and colleagues, one third of the patients will go on remission and will not experience any more subsequent episode, the second third of the patients will experience one or more psychotic episodes (stage 2), while the third group of patients will experience multiple relapses and unremitting illness which will be later described as chronic disorder (stage 3) [50].

3.3 Remission and relapse (stage 2)

Between stage 1 and 3 is the most heterogenous phase of the disorder, the remission and relapse stage. During this period of SSD, patients first experience a temporary or incomplete remission from the first episode, but then there is a relapse or even multiple relapses of psychotic symptoms in the form of episodes [10]. If looking at the chain of events in a chronological order, before being in remission, the patient first responses to the treatment, which is usually determined by a certain amount of reduction in symptoms (between 20–50%) on a validated rating scale such as the Positive and Negative Syndrome Scale (PANSS) or the Clinical Global Impression (CGI) [51, 52]. Then the patient moves to remission, which, according to the Remission in Schizophrenia Working Group (RSWG), is an "increasingly achievable stage in the treatment of schizophrenia, serving to expand the current ceiling of patient progress beyond "stability" [53]. Although there are various criteria on how remission is defined, it essentially means a period of the disorder when symptoms are mild and/or there is no "active" psychosis [53]. When symptoms start to reappear after this mild or symptom-free period, and the patient is experiencing a worsening in functioning, we are talking about relapse [54, 55]. Nonetheless, as mentioned previously, a third of patients might not relapse rather achieve recovery [50], a state where the patient is able to function both socially and occupationally and has considerable symptomatic improvement [55, 56].

The second stage of SSD is hence quite various in terms of the type and severity of symptoms. Nonetheless, in most cases, the negative and depressive / anxiety-like symptoms [25] are highly dominant in-between relapses, affecting the patient's quality of life enormously [57]. Throughout a relapse the positive and hostility-related symptoms might particularly increase [25, 55].

According to Fountoulakis and colleagues, the duration of this second phase is around 9 years on average, followed by a 13 years-long period dominated by depressive symptoms [25], so an up to 10-year long period for the second stage is adapted.

The primary treatment goal during this stage is first to achieve complete remission and then to prevent relapse as well as to stabilize the patient mediated by specialist care services [10]. Given the high level of negative and depressive/ anxiety-like symptoms, the secondary aim should be to alleviate these, either by using a novel second-generation antipsychotic medication such as cariprazine and amisulpride or a combination of antipsychotic and antidepressant medication [58].

3.4 Chronic psychosis (stage 3)

The third and final stage of the integrated staging model is the chronic psychosis stage. Throughout this period of the SSD the symptoms are still severe, persistent or unremitting [12]. The patients might continue to experience numerous relapses while usually suffering mostly from negative, affective (depressive/ anxiety-like) and neurocognitive symptoms, with the latter increasingly becoming the most prominent symptom group of the disorder over time [12, 25]. Suicidal ideation might also be more common at this stage of the illness [59]. Nonetheless, patients usually develop some kind of acceptance and integrate the fact of the disorder into their life [13].

The chronic psychosis stage of SSD begins about 15–20 years after the first episode [25, 45]. Patients in this late stage are usually disabled at a certain degree and are likely to be unemployed or retired [45].

Treatment in the chronic disorder stage is similar to stage 2 treatment with a high emphasis on the prevention of further exacerbation of the illness and long-term stabilization alongside with augmentation strategies and other psychosocial therapies such as active social participation and/or vocational rehabilitation [10]. Preferred pharmacological treatments include clozapine and long-acting antipsychotic medications [12], although drugs addressing negative and cognitive symptoms (such as cariprazine and amisulpride) may also be of benefit [58].

3.5 Summary of the integrated staging model

The integrated staging model starts with the prodrome (stage 0), which is a period of the SSD where patients are already experiencing some changes in their behavior alongside mild negative and affective symptoms (**Figure 10**). Diagnosis is usually not yet received as the symptoms are too mild and unspecific to be certain about what causes them. This period can last from a few weeks to years. Pharmacological interventions throughout the prodrome are still researched, nonetheless psychosocial therapies are thought to be beneficial.

The first stage of the SSD according to the integrated staging model is the onset of the first episode of psychosis characterized by positive and hostility-like symptoms. This period can last between 2 and 5 years in average. Regarding treatment, the emphasis is on alleviating mostly positive symptoms and stabilizing the patient.

The second stage is the remission and relapse stage which is the most heterogenous phase of the disorder. Throughout this period some patients might experience one or multiple relapses, however about a third of the patients will stay in remission and may go to recovery. The dominating symptoms in-between episodes are the negative and affective ones. The remission and relapse stage last about ten years, between the 5th and 15-20th year of the illness. The primary goal of treatment during this stage is the prevention of relapses and achieving complete remission and recovery.

The final stage of SSD is the chronic psychosis stage dominated by increasing neurocognitive symptoms. Patients arriving to this late stage are likely to be suffering from disability and unemployment. Alongside the pharmacological treatments that aim to prevent the further exacerbation of illness there is an emphasis on psychosocial therapies to increase the everyday functioning of patients.

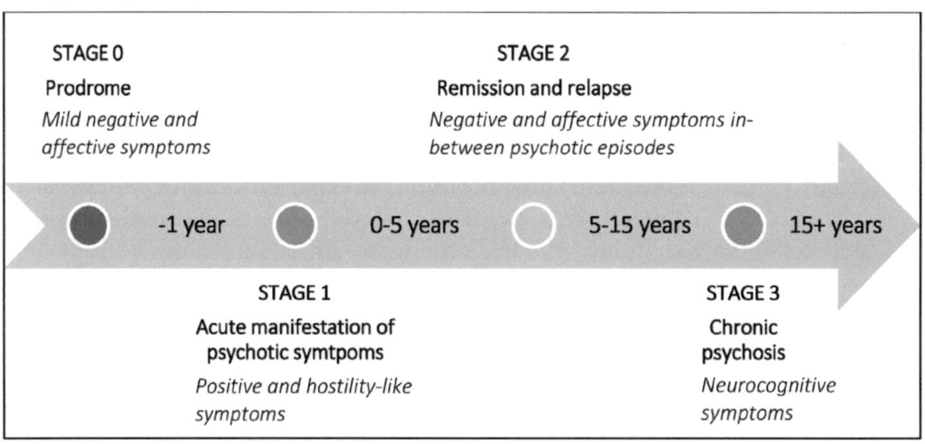

Figure 10.
The integrated staging model of schizophrenia spectrum disorders with timeline and symptom domains.

4. Conclusion

Clinical staging is a more refined form of diagnosis that provides information on how an illness progresses and where the patient lies within this progression [10]. It is based on the assumption that each stage can be described by a typical clinical profile with later stages being associated with greater symptom severity and that treating patients in the early stages of the disorder is more efficient [12]. The primary aim of introducing clinical staging into the field of psychiatry was to promote remission and recovery in the early stages of psychiatric disorders and hence to prevent patients to progress to later stages [10].

Since 1982, several staging concepts describing the course of psychiatric disorders have emerged. In this systematic review, we have identified and summarized 9 concepts that outline the clinical staging of schizophrenia spectrum disorders. Although there were some variations between the models, all identified the first episode of psychosis as a distinct stage that divides the course of the disorder into a *before* and *after* phase. Most of the variations in the concepts were due to the fact that there were disagreements in the number of stages before and after the first onset.

In order to unify the described concepts an integrated staging model of schizophrenia spectrum disorder has emerged that describes the course of SSD in four stages; the prodrome (stage 0), the onset (stage 1), remission and relapse (stage 2) and chronic psychosis (stage 3). The integrated model also provides timeline around when patients are likely to enter the next stage as well as what symptoms dominate and how to best treat them. Nonetheless, it is also important to note that not all patients will go through all stages and the primary goal of any treatment is to prevent patients to enter a later stage.

Conflict of interest

All authors are co-workers of Gedeon Richter Plc.

Author details

Zsófia Borbála Dombi*, Ágota Barabássy, Barbara Sebe, István Laszlovszky and György Németh
Gedeon Richter Plc., Budapest, Hungary

*Address all correspondence to: dombizsb@richter.hu

References

[1] American Psychiatric Association. American Psychiatric Association: Diagnostic and Statistical Manual of Mental Disorders Fifth Edition. Arlington. 2013.

[2] Bhati MT. Defining psychosis: The evolution of DSM-5 schizophrenia spectrum disorders. Curr Psychiatry Rep. 2013;15(409).

[3] Guloksuz S, Van Os J. The slow death of the concept of schizophrenia and the painful birth of the psychosis spectrum. Psychol Med. 2018;48(2):229-244.

[4] Adam D. On the spectrum. Nature. 2013;496.

[5] John M, Sukanta S, David C, Joy W. Schizophrenia: A concise overview of incidence, prevalence, and mortality. Epidemiol Rev. 2008;30(1):67-76.

[6] Orrico-Sánchez A, López-Lacort M, Munõz-Quiles C, Sanfélix-Gimeno G, Diéz-Domingo J. Epidemiology of schizophrenia and its management over 8-years period using real-world data in Spain. BMC Psychiatry. 2020;20(149).

[7] WHO. WHO | Schizophrenia. Schizophrenia. 2018.

[8] Perälä J, Suvisaari J, Saarni SI, Kuoppasalmi K, Isometsä E, Pirkola S, et al. Lifetime prevalence of psychotic and bipolar I disorders in a general population. Arch Gen Psychiatry. 2007;64:19-28.

[9] Os J van. "Schizophrenia" does not exist. BMJ. 2016;352:i375.

[10] McGorry PD, Nelson B, Goldstone S, Yung AR. Clinical staging: A heuristic and practical strategy for new research and better health and social outcomes for psychotic and related mood disorders. Canadian Journal of Psychiatry. 2010.

[11] Cosci F, Fava GA. Staging of mental disorders: Systematic review. Psychother Psychosom. 2013;82:20-34.

[12] Agius M, Goh C, Ulhaq S, McGorry P. The staging model in schizophrenia, and its clinical implications. Psychiatr Danub. 2010;22:211-2020.

[13] Hoffman BF. The stages of schizophrenia and their management. Can Fam physician. 1982;28:2046-2050.

[14] Dave S, Boardman J. Person-centered care in psychiatric practice. Indian J Soc Psychiatry. 2018;34(4):333-336.

[15] Fava GA, Kellner R. Staging: A neglected dimension in psychiatric classification. Acta Psychiatr Scand. 1993;87:225-230.

[16] Lieberman JA, Perkins D, Belger A, Chakos M, Jarskog F, Boteva K, et al. The early stages of schizophrenia: Speculations on pathogenesis, pathophysiology, and therapeutic approaches. Biol Psychiatry. 2001;50:884-897.

[17] Insel TR. Rethinking schizophrenia. Nature. 2010;468(188):187-193.

[18] Khamker N. First episode schizophrenia. South African Fam Pract. 2015;57(5):29-33.

[19] Singh SP, Cooper JE, Fisher HL, Tarrant CJ, Lloyd T, Banjo J, et al. Determining the chronology and components of psychosis onset: The Nottingham onset schedule (NOS). Schizophr Res. 2005;80:117-130.

[20] Godin O, Fond G, Bulzacka E, Schürhoff F, Boyer L, Myrtille A, et al. Validation and refinement of the clinical staging model in a French cohort of outpatient with schizophrenia

(FACE-SZ). Prog Neuro-Psychopharmacology Biol Psychiatry. 2019;92:226-234.

[21] Berendsen S, van der Paardt JW, Van HL, van Bruggen M, Nusselder H, Jalink M, et al. Staging and profiling for schizophrenia spectrum disorders: Inter-rater reliability after a short training course. Prog Neuro-Psychopharmacology Biol Psychiatry. 2020;99:109856.

[22] Addington J, Liu L, Goldstein BI, Wang J, Kennedy SH, Bray S, et al. Clinical staging for youth at-risk for serious mental illness. Early Interv Psychiatry. 2020;1-9.

[23] Griffa A, Baumann PS, Klauser P, Mullier E, Cleusix M, Jenni R, et al. Brain connectivity alterations in early psychosis: from clinical to neuroimaging staging. Transl Psychiatry. 2019;9(62).

[24] Lee TY, Kim M, Kim SN, Kwon JS. Reconsidering clinical staging model: A case of genetic high risk for schizophrenia. Psychiatry Investig. 2017;14(1):107-109.

[25] Fountoulakis KN, Dragioti E, Theofilidis AT, Wikilund T, Atmatzidis X, Nimatoudis I, et al. Staging of schizophrenia with the use of PANSS: An international multi-center study. Int J Neuropsychopharmacol. 2019;22(11):681-697.

[26] Wood SJ, Yung AR, McGorry PD, Pantelis C. Neuroimaging and treatment evidence for clinical staging in psychotic disorders: From the at-risk mental state to chronic schizophrenia. Biological Psychiatry. 2011.

[27] Mathalon DH. Challenges associated with application of clinical staging models to psychotic disorders. Biol Psychiatry. 2011;70(7):600-601.

[28] Cornblatt B, Lencz T, Obuchowski M. The schizophrenia prodrome: Treatment and high-risk perspectives. Schizophr Res. 2002;54:177-186.

[29] Addington J. The prodromal stage of psychotic illness: Observation, detection or intervention? J Psychiatry Neurosci. 2003;28(2):93-97.

[30] Conroy SK, Francis MM, Hulvershorn LA. Identifying and treating the prodromal phases of bipolar disorder and schizophrenia. Curr Treat Options Psychiatry. 2018;5(1):113-128.

[31] Buehlmann E, Berger GE, Aston J, Gschwandtner U, Pflueger MO, Borgwardt SJ, et al. Hippocampus abnormalities in at risk mental states for psychosis? A cross-sectional high resolution region of interest magnetic resonance imaging study. J Psychiatr Res. 2010;44(7):447-453.

[32] Jung WH, Kim JS, Jang JH, Choi JS, Jung MH, Park JY, et al. Cortical thickness reduction in individuals at ultra-high-risk for psychosis. Schizophr Bull. 2011;37(4):839-849.

[33] Fusar-Poli P, Broome MR, Woolley JB, Johns LC, Tabraham P, Bramon E, et al. Altered brain function directly related to structural abnormalities in people at ultra high risk of psychosis: Longitudinal VBM-fMRI study. J Psychiatr Res. 2011;45(2):190-198.

[34] D. Howes O, Fusar-Poli P, Bloomfield M, Selvaraj S, McGuire P. From the Prodrome to chronic schizophrenia: The neurobiology underlying psychotic symptoms and cognitive impairments. Curr Pharm Des. 2012;18(4):459-465.

[35] Cornblatt BA, Lencz T, Kane JM. Treatment of the schizophrenia prodrome: Is it presently ethical? Schizophr Res. 2001;51:31-38.

[36] McGuire P, Selvaraj S, Howes O. Is clinical intervention in the ultra high

risk phase effective? Rev Bras Psiquiatr. 2011;33(Supl II).

[37] Yung AR, Phillips LJ, McGorry PD, McFarlane CA, Francey S, Harrigan S, et al. Prediction of psychosis. A step towards indicated prevention of schizophrenia. Br J Psychiatry Suppl. 1998;172(33):14-20.

[38] McGorry PD, Yung AR, Phillips LJ, Yuen HP, Francey S, Cosgrave EM, et al. Randomized controlled trial of interventions designed to reduce the risk of progression to first-episode psychosis in a clinical sample with subthreshold symptoms. Arch Gen Psychiatry. 2002;59(10):921-928.

[39] McGlashan TH, Zipursky RB, Perkins D, Addington J, Miller T, Woods SW, et al. Randomized, double-blind trial of olanzapine versus placebo in patients prodromally symptomatic for psychosis. Am J Psychiatry. 2006;163:790-799.

[40] Schmidt SJ, Schultze-Lutter F, Schimmelmann BG, Maric NP, Salokangas RKR, Riecher-Rössler A, et al. EPA guidance on the early intervention in clinical high risk states of psychoses. Eur Psychiatry. 2015;30(3):388-404.

[41] Agius M, Butler S, Holt C. Does early diagnosis and treatment of schizophrenia lead to improved long-term outcomes? Neuropsychiatry (London). 2011;1(6):553-565.

[42] Roberts J, Gracia Canales A, Blanthorn-Hazell S, Craciun Boldeanu A, Judge D. Characterizing the experience of agitation in patients with bipolar disorder and schizophrenia. BMC Psychiatry. 2018;18(104).

[43] Breitborde NJK, Srihari VH, Woods SW. Review of the operational definition for first-episode psychosis. Early Interv Psychiatry. 2009;3(4): 259-265.

[44] McGlashan TH. A selective review of recent north American long-term followup studies of schizophrenia. Schizophr Bull. 1988;14:515-542.

[45] Costa LG, Massuda R, Pedrini M, Passos IC, Czepielewski LS, Brietzke E, et al. Functioning in early and late stages of schizophrenia. Trends Psychiatry Psychother. 2014;36(4):209-213.

[46] Wyatt RJ. Neuroleptics and the natural course of schizophrenia. Schizophr Bull. 1991;17(2):325-351.

[47] Patel MX, De Zoysa N, Bernadt M, David A. Depot and oral antipsychotics: Patient preferences and attitudes are not the same thing. J Psychopharmacol. 2009;23(7):789-796.

[48] Johnson DAW, Freeman H. Drug defaulting by patients on long-acting phenothiazines. Psychol Med. 1973;3(1):115-119.

[49] Miller BJ. A review of second-generation antipsychotic discontinuation in first-episode psychosis. J Psychiatr Pract. 2008;14(5):289-300.

[50] Shepherd M, Watt D, Falloon I, Smeeton N. The natural history of schizophrenia: A five-year follow-up study of outcome and prediction in a representative sample of schizophrenics. Psychol Med Monogr Suppl. 1989;15:1-46.

[51] Leucht S, Kane JM, Kissling W, Hamann J, Etschel E, Engel R. Clinical implications of brief psychiatric rating scale scores. Br J Psychiatry. 2005;187:366-371.

[52] Correll CU, Kishimoto T, Nielsen J, Kane JM. Quantifying clinical relevance in the treatment of schizophrenia. Clin Ther. 2011;33:B16–B39.

[53] Andreasen NC, Carpenter WT, Kane JM, Lasser RA, Marder SR,

Weinberger DR. Remission in schizophrenia: Proposed criteria and rationale for consensus Nancy. Am J Psychiatry. 2005;162:441-449.

[54] San L, Serrano M, Cañas F, Romero SL, Sánchez-Cabezudo Á, Villar M. Towards a pragmatic and operational definition of relapse in schizophrenia: A Delphi consensus approach. Int J Psychiatry Clin Pract. 2015;19:90-98.

[55] Lee BJ, Kim SW, Kim JJ, Yu JC, Lee KY, Won SH, et al. Defining treatment response, remission, relapse, and recovery in first-episode psychosis: A survey among Korean experts. Psychiatry Investig. 2020;17(2):163-174.

[56] Menezes NM, Arenovich T, Zipursky RB. A systematic review of longitudinal outcome studies of first-episode psychosis. Psychol Med. 2006;36:1349-1362.

[57] Novick D, Montgomery W, Cheng Y, Moneta V, Haro JM. Impact of negative symptoms on quality of life in patients with schizophrenia. Value Heal. 2015;18(7):A836–A837.

[58] Cerveri G, Gesi C, Mencacci C. Pharmacological treatment of negative symptoms in schizophrenia: Update and proposal of a clinical algorithm. Neuropsychiatr Dis Treat. 2019;15:1525-1535.

[59] Roy A. Suicide in chronic schizophrenia. Br J Psychiatry. 1982;141(2):171-177.

Chapter 4

The Many Faces of Negative Symptoms in Schizophrenia

Mihaela Fadgyas Stanculete and Octavia Capatina

Abstract

Negative symptoms are relatively frequent across schizophrenia spectrum disorders diagnostic categories and they represent deficits in different domains such as emotional, volitional and experiential. Even though negative symptoms have long been recognized as a core feature of schizophrenia, their definition has been changing over time. Different conceptualization classified this category of symptoms as primary or secondary, persistent or transient. At the current moment there are five agreed upon domains of the concept of negative symptoms, which are separated into two dimensions—experience (anhedonia, avolition, asociality) and expression (blunted affect, alogia). Multiple mechanistic pathways have been proposed and investigated for each dimension and for each domain. The current chapter attempts to address recent advances in the literature regarding the concepts, definitions and classifications of negative symptoms and their etiological model.

Keywords: anhedonia, avolition, alogia, blunted affect, negative symptoms, schizophrenia

1. Introduction

Schizophrenia is a chronic, debilitating disorder that affects approximately 1% of the world's population [1]. The disorder is a significant socioeconomic burden because of the early onset of the disease, the low remission rates, and their debilitating consequences: as the disease's progression leads to the inability, for a significant share of schizophrenic patients, to fulfill their professional, social and household roles [2]. Phenomenologically schizophrenia is considered to be a heterogeneous syndrome including several dimensions: positive, disorganization, cognitive, affective, and negative dimension. These are the most commonly reported by factor analytic studies dimensions of schizophrenia [3–5].

Negative symptoms have long been recognized as a core feature of schizophrenia, and the current studies report that their severity has a more significant impact on real-world functioning and quality of life than other categories of symptoms [6–10]. Negative symptoms, by their definition, interfere with the patient's ability to maintain social activities or personal relationships, to work or study, and even to live independently and are minimally influenced by antipsychotic medication [11–13]. Even though the attention has shifted from the positive to the negative symptoms in the last decades, the latter still represent an unmet therapeutical target, and very few pharmaceutical agents are labeling indications for negative symptoms [14–17].

Negative symptoms have been commonly described as first symptoms of schizophrenia, and very frequently, they appear during the prodromal phase of the disorder [18, 19]. The prevalence of negative symptoms is hard to establish, with reports from literature ranging between 40% and 90%, these differences result from the heterogeneity of the used definitions, constitutive factors, and assessment methods [20]. The European First Episode Schizophrenia Trial reported that at least one negative symptom was noted in up to 54.2% of the patients at baseline [21]. The Clinical Antipsychotic Trials of Interventions Effectiveness, which is one of the most extensive controlled studies for schizophrenia, reported negative symptoms in 40% of the patients [22], and the CLAMORS study reported one or more negative symptoms were present in 57.6% of patients [23]. What is known is that they can occur at any point during the illness, but the long-term course is less clear. Some studies report stability of negative domain [24], while others describe an unstable course [25]. Many factors could be accountable for this difference, but it is widely accepted that improvement in negative symptoms is more common during the first years of the disorder, and an exacerbation is frequently seen in chronic patients [26].

Across studies, it is generally evidenced that negative symptoms are frequently reported in any disease phase. They are associated with poor functional outcomes, which is why it is imperative to assess and address these symptoms to improve the quality of life for patients with schizophrenia.

2. The concept of negative symptoms in schizophrenia

2.1 Early descriptions

The classification of the symptoms of schizophrenia as being positive or negative regards the fact that positive symptoms are a surplus to normal experiences, for example, hallucinations or delusions, whereas the negative symptoms are represented by diminished experiences or expression [27]. The term of negative symptoms was borrowed from neurology, and it was coined by John Reynolds in 1858 and was introduced in psychiatry by the French psychiatrists Gaetan Gatian de Clerambault and Henry Ey [28].

The negative symptoms were considered a fundamental feature of the disease since its first descriptions by Emil Kraepelin and Eugen Bleuler [27]. Emil Kraepelin, influenced by the work of Alois Alzheimer, was the one who named the disease dementia praecox. He considered that the process underpinning the manifestation of the disease was an affective degeneration. In his treatise "Dementia praecox and paraphrenia", he described the flat affect and the motivational deficits, which are now called negative symptoms, and he proposed the theory that the affective deficit represents the basis for the psychopathological process [27–30].

Eugen Bleuler renamed the disease schizophrenia and emphasized that there is a group of disorders under this name. At a descriptive level, he introduces a dichotomy between the symptoms of schizophrenia, and he labels the fundamental and accessory symptoms. The fundamental symptoms are described as the essence of the illness necessary to diagnose loose associations, ambivalence, affective flattening, and avolition. The accessory symptoms are hallucinations and delusions that were not necessary to diagnose schizophrenia but were highly visible and often the reason for clinical presentation. Unlike his predecessor, he considers that the affect as a process is intact in schizophrenia and that the fundamental psychopathological process is the splitting between affect and cognition, from which the symptoms of the disease arise [27, 28, 30].

The interest for negative symptoms decreased and shifted towards the positive symptoms once Chlorpromazine was developed and introduced in psychiatric wards in 1952. The awareness regarding the importance of these symptoms reemerged in the last decades because of their negative influence on the patients' real-life function [10, 11, 31].

2.2 Current perspective

The interest for the negative symptoms is constantly growing, although it has been about 40 years since Nancy Andreasen and co-workers (1982) resumed this research area and highlighted the importance of this category of symptoms. Andreasen defined twenty negative symptoms, which were grouped into five factors: flat affect, alogia, avolition/apathy, anhedonia/social withdrawal, and attention deficit. She proposed that negative and positive symptoms are part of a continuum representing the extreme and opposite poles of this continuum. Patients presenting mixed symptoms, positive and negative symptoms, were considered intermediate patients [28, 32].

Later, Timothy Crow [33] postulated the hypothesis of two types of disease, schizophrenia type I and type II. Type I is characterized by positive symptoms (hallucinations, delusions), showing a good response to neuroleptic medication, without intellectual deficit, and with an increase in D2 receptors. Type II is characterized by negative symptoms (alogia, affective flattening, decreased interest, and pleasure), an inadequate response to neuroleptic medication, intellectual deficits, and changes in the temporal lobes' neural structures. According to this author, type I could develop negative symptoms and progress to type II, but type II could not transform into type I, even though positive symptoms could appear [33].

In 1988 William Carpenter and collaborators brought to attention a new perspective on the concept of negative symptoms and made an essential distinction between idiopathic, primary negative symptoms and secondary negative symptoms. Secondary negative symptoms occur as side effects of neuroleptic medication (extrapyramidal symptoms, sedation) or secondary to depression, social deprivation or substimulation or secondary to positive symptoms (active social withdrawal secondary to paranoid ideation, or diminished expression, which could be a coping strategy for patients in an acute psychotic episode who are unable to process tumultuous hallucinations). At a phenomenological level, primary and secondary negative are very similar and yet very hard to distinguish. The diagnosis of primary negative symptoms, according to Carpenter, should be only a diagnosis of exclusion. The importance of distinguishing these categories of symptoms is that secondary negative symptoms may be responsive to specific treatments [34].

As a result of this classification, deficit schizophrenia was introduced to define patients with primary and persistent negative symptoms. The dichotomy, deficit/non-deficit schizophrenia, is based exclusively on the presence or absence of primary and stable negative symptoms [34]. The diagnostic criteria for deficit schizophrenia are presented in **Table 1**. Several subsequent studies have compared patients with deficit schizophrenia versus non-deficit schizophrenia and found overwhelming evidence that the two types are different in that concerns risk factors, premorbid functioning, disease evolution, neurobiological basis, and response to treatment. The clinical picture of deficit schizophrenia shows more significant social withdrawal, anergia, more severe cognitive impairments, poorer premorbid adjustment than non-deficit schizophrenia, and often summer birth instead of non-deficit schizophrenia, which predominates winter birth [37–41]. Although the two diagnostic categories have been validated in several studies, the evolution over time of negative symptoms does not always allow a clear distinction between

a. The presence of at least two of the following six negative symptoms: i. Decreased emotional expression (observed behavior); ii. Affective flattening (e.g. a narrow range of the patient's subjective emotional experience); iii. Alogia; iv. Diminished interests; v. Diminished goals; vi. Diminished social interest;
b. The presence of symptoms described in point (a) for at least 12 months including periods of clinical stability;
c. The symptoms described at point (a) are primary symptoms, not secondary to other factors such as anxiety, medication side effects, psychotic symptoms, intellectual disability or depression;
d. The patient meets the DSM criteria (3rd edition, or later editions) for schizophrenia.

Table 1.
Diagnostic criteria for deficit schizophrenia [34–36].

primary and secondary symptoms, making the diagnosis very difficult. Moreover, first psychotic episode patients represent another diagnostical challenge [42–44].

A different approach, which tried to reduce the heterogeneity of negative symptoms, was proposed by the National Institute for Mental Health (USA) in The Consensus Statement on Negative Symptoms (2006), which defined the constitutive factors of the negative domain: flat affect, alogia, social withdrawal, avolition, and anhedonia, essentially the same areas that have been defined by Nancy Andreasen (1982) except for the attention deficit. A short definition of each symptom, according to this consensus, is presented in **Table 2** [45].

As a result of the same consensus, the National Institute for mental Health defined the concept of persistent negative symptoms, which is more applicable in the clinical setting than the concept of deficit schizophrenia because of its more permissive criteria. The criteria for the persistent negative symptoms imply only a period of six months, with at least moderate intensity negative symptoms and low levels of positive, depressive, and extrapyramidal symptoms. Secondary negative symptoms can be included in this category if they are not responsive to a specific treatment [45].

In the attempt to describe the nature, the etiology, and find operational criteria for research in the field, other specific terms were defined: predominant, prominent, enduring/non-enduring negative symptoms. Unfortunately, there is

Flat affect	A decrease in the expression of emotions and emotional reactivity to events, observed spontaneously during speech or after targeted questions (facial expression, intonation, and gestures)
Alogia	Quantitative reduction of speech and spontaneity (the amount of information spontaneously developed by the patient in addition to the necessary answers to the questions).
Social withdrawal	Interactions and initiatives to have social contacts are diminished due to decreased motivation and decreased desire to form or maintain relationships with other people.
Anhedonia	Diminished experience of pleasure for a variety of activities or events, over time of the activities or events (consumer anhedonia) or for subsequent activities and events (anticipatory anhedonia)
Avolition	Reducing the initiative and persistence of goal-oriented activities due to diminished motivation

Table 2.
Definition of negative symptoms of schizophrenia [45].

no consensus regarding the exact definition of any of these terms as they were only used for research purposes [9].

Up to the present point, negative symptoms are considered to represent a heterogeneous domain of psychopathology. Recent factor analytic studies have provided evidence that the domain of negative symptoms can be grouped into two factors: avolition/apathy and diminished expression. The apathy/avolition subdomain includes avolition, social withdrawal, and anhedonia, and the diminished expression includes affective flattening and alogia [46–48]. This factorial structure has been confirmed by several studies using different scales for the evaluation of negative symptoms: Scale for the Assessment of Negative Symptoms (SANS), Positive and Negative Syndrome Scale (PANSS), Negative Symptoms Assessment Scale (NSA-16) and more recently developed scales Clinical Assessment Interview for Negative Symptoms (CAINS) and Brief Negative Symptom Scale (BNSS), which were specially developed to evaluate this factorial structure [49, 50]. Several studies have compared the importance of these domains regarding clinical features, disease progression, and impact on functioning. The domain of diminished expression (DE) turned out to be more persistent over time, have a higher prevalence in the early stages of the disease, and be associated with a longer duration of the prodromal phase of the disease than the apathy/avolition (AA) [51–53]. The AA domain is associated with poorer functioning, with a longer duration of untreated psychosis and non-adherence to treatment. These associations were not reported for the DE domain [47, 52, 54]. Research up to this point provided evidence that the AA and DE domains represent different clinical aspects of schizophrenia. Moreover, if these areas have different etiologies and should be approached differently from a therapeutic point of view are elements in an ongoing investigation, neuroimaging studies currently support this hypothesis [8, 55].

To date, no consensus has been reached on how to approach negative symptoms: categorical versus dimensional. Numerous studies demonstrated the validity of deficit schizophrenia construct or the subtype characterized by primary and persistent negative symptoms [51, 52, 54]. However, the dimensional approach is supported by several studies that have shown the presence of negative symptoms in other disorders than schizophrenia, such as schizoaffective disorder, depression, Parkinson's disease, Huntington's disease, Alzheimer's disease, temporal lobe epilepsy, and even in the general population [8, 55, 56].

3. The neurobiology of negative symptoms in schizophrenia

The heterogeneity in etiology and clinical manifestation of the negative symptoms in schizophrenia led to the exploration of several structural abnormalities, pathways, and mechanisms which may underlie this complex of symptoms. The attempt to reduce these symptoms' heterogeneity leads to concepts of deficit and non-deficit schizophrenia and diminished expression and avolition/apathy domains. Different hypotheses have been constructed for these models' pathophysiological mechanisms, but unfortunately without fully satisfying results [8, 9, 55, 56].

3.1 Deficit schizophrenia versus non-deficit schizophrenia

After deficit schizophrenia was described, several studies brought out data supporting the hypothesis that deficit schizophrenia differs from non-deficit schizophrenia in terms of risk factors, premorbid functioning, the evolution of the disease, neurobiological basis, and response to treatment [37–41]. Epidemiological studies support a prevalence of deficit schizophrenia: 15% of patients with a first episode of the disease, 25–30% in clinical trials, and 14–17% in population studies [37, 57, 58]. Structural and functional brain imaging studies have highlighted several differences between patients with deficit and non-deficit schizophrenia. Abnormalities and asymmetries in the temporal lobe level, cerebrospinal fluid accumulations in the left temporal lobe, volume reduction of the right temporal lobe have been reported in patients with deficit schizophrenia compared with patients with non-deficit schizophrenia and healthy subjects. Both groups of patients had a reduced volume of the dorsolateral prefrontal cortex and temporal lobes than healthy subjects [59, 60]. Several studies have reported white matter abnormalities, especially in the frontoparietal and frontotemporal circuits in patients with deficit schizophrenia. These patients present discontinuities in the inferior longitudinal fasciculus, arcuate fasciculus, and uncinate fasciculus, and it has been suggested that there may be a connection between these structural changes and the social and emotional dysfunctions characteristic for deficit schizophrenia [59, 60]. Functional imaging investigations report a decrease in glucose metabolism and a decrease in the frontal and parietal lobes' blood flow in cases of deficit schizophrenia versus non-deficit schizophrenia or healthy volunteers [61, 62]. Studies that used functional MRI to assess the response to the reward reported a reduction of dorsal caudate nucleus activity in patients with deficit schizophrenia [63, 64].

Regarding the treatment of deficit schizophrenia, respectively of primary negative symptoms, the efficacy of several antipsychotics was evaluated: clozapine, olanzapine, zotepine, and amisulpride. These therapeutic options are superior to placebo therapy and first-generation antipsychotics, but not other classes of atypical antipsychotics, data suggesting that they would be effective for secondary negative symptoms [65–68]. Recent studies have evaluated the efficacy of add-on therapies with agents that stimulate NMDA receptors: glycine, D-serine, and D-cycloserine, but no significant improvement in symptoms was reported on the primary negative ones [15, 40, 69, 70].

3.2 Persistent negative symptoms

Persistent negative symptoms are a looser category than deficit schizophrenia as potential causes of secondary negative symptoms are not completely ruled out, but it is assumed that the secondary negative symptoms' clinical expression is mild [45]. Also, this category includes all negative symptoms, primary or secondary, that do not respond to commonly used treatments, which are apparent during periods of clinical stability of the disease and interfere with the patient's functionality [45]. There is great variability in the prevalence of persistent negative symptoms due to different definitions used for this category. Prevalence of persistent negative symptoms are higher than deficit schizophrenia and were estimated between 35% and 60% [21, 71–73].

Structural and functional imaging studies have reported volume reduction of the gray matter in the temporal lobes, cortical atrophy of the right superior temporal gyrus, right parahippocampal gyrus, and left orbitofrontal gyrus, and that structural abnormality of the white matter in the frontal lobes could be associated with persistent negative symptoms [74–77].

Dopaminergic antagonism is the only common mechanism of drugs used to treat psychosis. However, subcortical dopamine excess is accompanied by a prefrontal dopaminergic function, which encompasses a reduced D1 receptor activation in the prefrontal cortex, dopamine hypoactivity in the caudate nucleus, and modifications in D3 receptor activity. These alterations appear to contribute to the pathogenesis of negative symptoms. Cariprazine is an atypical antipsychotic that is a partial agonist of dopamine receptors D3 and D2, with high selectivity for D3 receptors, which have been shown to be effective for predominant negative symptoms [78, 79]. Another compound, MIN-101, that has no affinity for dopaminergic receptors and acts on sigma-2 and serotonergic receptors 5-HT2A effectively reduces persistent negative symptoms [80].

3.3 Negative symptoms domains: avolition/apathy and diminished expression

Factor analysis studies have suggested that negative symptoms include two domains: apathy/avolition and diminished expression, which led to building separate hypotheses for these domains [45, 47, 52]. In current conceptualizations, the avolition/apathy domain is defined as deficits in different motivation areas. Two possible mechanisms and circuits are considered to be involved: the reward circuit and the salience circuit [81]. Functional MRI studies tried to elucidate the substrate of the motivational deficit using tasks involving reward anticipation, and it was found that there is an association between the activation of the ventral striatum and the apathy/avolition domain. This relationship has not been confirmed for the diminished expression domain. Only a limited number of studies have investigated the correlations between neural structures and the apathy/avolition domain, and the following results were reported: a low volume of the frontal lobes, thinning of the anterior cingulate cortex and orbitofrontal cortex, and structural abnormalities of connectivity between the medial orbitofrontal cortex and the anterior rostral cingulate cortex [55, 82–85].

Cognitive-behavioral therapy was the first form of alternative therapy targeting poor motivation, anhedonia, and irrational cognitions. It promotes the patient's involvement in defining goals and aims and targets, improving functionality and recovery of the patients. A positive effect of cognitive-behavioral therapy on negative symptoms in combination with antipsychotic medication has been proved, and the beneficial effects persist even after stopping therapy. Functional changes, highlighted by functional brain imaging studies, at striatal levels underlie this type of therapy's effectiveness [86, 87].

Some studies suggest that dopaminergic agonists: methylphenidate, amphetamine, lisdexamfetamine, modafinil, selegiline are involved in relieving negative symptoms without worsening the positive symptoms. The exact mechanisms by which this class acts are not completely elucidated. Increasing dopamine and noradrenaline at the frontocortical level or the dopamine action at the striatal limbic level are possible mechanisms involved in the assumed action of dopaminergic agonists on a motivational deficit [17, 55, 88].

The inflammatory hypothesis of schizophrenia suggests that alterations in the prenatal immune system are involved in the disease's etiology. Anti-inflammatory agents studied so far are pregnenolone, acetylsalicylic acid, cyclooxygenase-2, minocycline, N-acetylcysteine, and omega-3 fatty acids. To date, clinical trials have seemed promising, but these studies need to be replicated on a larger scale [89–92].

High frequency transcranial magnetic stimulation ($\leq$10 Hz) intensifies metabolism and excitability in the prefrontal cortex. It has been proved to be effective in treating negative symptoms when applied in the early stages of schizophrenia. The mechanisms of action of this method involve modulation of NDMA receptors and striatal dopamine release. This technique has not been proven effective for alogia, but only for the other negative symptoms [93, 94].

Transcranial direct current stimulation has been mainly studied for positive symptoms, auditory hallucinations, but an improvement of negative symptoms as a subsidiary result, especially motivational deficits, has been reported. The modulation of cortical–subcortical networks can explain the benefits for negative symptoms [95, 96].

The diminished expression domain's pathophysiological mechanisms have received less attention than those involved in the apathy/avolition domain. It has been hypothesized that this domain is correlated with neurocognitive deficits and social cognition deficits [97]. In treatment naïve patients, there is an association between expressive deficits and neurological soft signs, which suggests the existence of diffuse neurodevelopmental abnormalities. Functional neuroimaging studies that investigated impaired emotional processing have shown a hypoactivity of different neural networks: the prefrontal, ventrolateral cortex, the amygdala, cingulate cortex, and the cuneus [98–100]. Activation of the anterior rostral cingulate cortex was negatively correlated with the diminished expression domain in the tasks which involve an interaction between reward and cognition [101].

Cognitive training, which aims to improve neurocognitive skills and social cognition, has been shown to restore the disrupted neural networks in the prefrontal cortex and anterior rostral cingulate cortex [102].

Social skills training for emotion perception, recognition, and expression, aims to educate patients about the necessity of social skills, verbal and nonverbal communication improvement, and it has been shown that it facilitates the release of oxytocin [103]. Considering the hypothesis that the strengthening social cognition could have beneficial effects on the diminished expression, the administration of intranasal oxytocin was studied, given its action on serotonin and dopamine in the nucleus accumbens and amygdala. Oxytocin is effective in emotion recognition and the theory of mind as add-on therapy and being used in the long term [104].

4. Genetic basis of negative symptoms

The progress in the genetics of schizophrenia in the last years has been noticeable. Heritability represents a statistical estimate to quantitate the relative genetic contribution to a trait relative to its environmental contributors. Heritability is the amount or proportion of phenotypic variance of the disease of interest in the population that is inherited through genetic factors. The heritability of schizophrenia has been established at 81% [105], making the genetic factor the most significant for the disease.

According to evidence from previous family and association studies, it has been suggested that genetic factors are involved in the development of schizophrenia and also in its clinical presentation. Studies that investigated genes potentially involved in negative symptoms pathogenesis highlighted that classifying patients with schizophrenia into specific subtypes based on predominant symptoms is useful for selecting the specific treatment. The findings, and references for these studies are summarized on **Table 3**.

Genetics is rapidly growing, with technological discoveries making it increasingly possible to identify common and rare variants on genomic DNA. Much new and confirmatory work remains to be performed to elucidate the role of specific genetic variants in negative symptoms development and the distinct ways the genes and environment interact to result in schizophrenia susceptibility.

Author	Year	Findings	Journal
Fanous et al.	2005	Variation in DTNBP1 may predispose subjects to a form of schizophrenia with high levels of negative symptoms.	American Journal of Psychiatry [106]
DeRosse et al.	2006	Significant association between the CTCTAC haplotype and lifetime severity of negative symptoms in patients with schizophrenia.	American Journal of Psychiatry [107]
Pelayo-Terán et al.	2008	Patients with a Val158 homozygote genotype had a higher severity of negative symptoms at the onset of the schizophrenia	American Journal of Medical Genetics [108]
Wessman et al.	2009	DTNBP1 gene is associated with a schizophrenia phenotype characterized by prominent negative symptoms	Biological Psychiatry [109]
Bertolino et al.	2009	Negative symptoms were weakly associated with promoter rs1236428	Brain [110]
Petrovsky et al.	2010	Association of prepulse inhibition deficits and polymorphisms in the a3 subunits of the CHRNA gene cluster. CHRNA3 polymorphisms were also associated with negative symptoms	Neuropsychopharmacology [111]
Xu et al.	2013	Common genetic variations (ST3GAL1, RNF144, CTNNA3 and ZNF385D) are associated with negative symptoms of schizophrenia using meta-analysis.	PloS one [112]
Mezquida et al.	2016	BDNF Val66Met polymorphism is associated with negative symptoms severity	European Psychiatry [113]
Edwards et al.	2016	NKAIN2 was significantly associated with negative symptoms	Schizophrenia bulletin [114]
Gao et al.	2018	Abnormal peripheral gene expression DNA methylation of MMP9 possible biomarker for negative symptom	Frontiers in Genetics [115]
Schneider et al.	2019	Negative symptoms are core manifestations of psychosis in individuals with 22q11DS that strongly impact global functioning.	Schizophrenia Research [116]

Abbreviations: DTNBP1 (dystrobrevin binding protein 1), CHRNA3 (nicotinic acetylcholine receptor), BDNF (brain-derived neurotrophic factor), MMP9 (Matrix metalloproteinase-9), NKAIN2 (Sodium/Potassium Transporting ATPase Interacting 2), 22q11DS (22q11 deletion syndrome).

Table 3.
Genes potentially involved in negative symptoms' pathogenesis.

5. Conclusions

Conceptual work has highlighted that negative symptoms can be defined as primary or secondary, persistent, or transient, and they encompass two distinct domains: avolition/apathy and diminished expression. Deficit schizophrenia is defined as primary enduring negative symptoms, but more operative for research and clinical setting is the concept of persistent negative symptoms. Considering the heterogeneity of negative symptoms has brought some progress in research on their genetic and neurobiological basis and treatment approaches. Unfortunately, their underlying pathophysiology is still unknown, and the treatment remains a critical unmet need.

Several hypotheses have been proposed for the pathophysiology of schizophrenia, from which the dopaminergic hypothesis remains the leading one. The dopaminergic hypofunction of the frontal lobe and the mesolimbic structures seems to be underlying the negative symptoms. Despite the advances in the field, many clinical trials still consider the negative symptoms as a monolithic construct which might be the reason for the unsatisfactory results.

Further research directions should concentrate on the two distinct negative symptoms dimensions apathy/avolition and diminished expression, and even further on each symptom and its pathophysiology. Another interesting approach is the transdiagnostic one, which could be helpful in the attempt to disentangle the mechanisms underlying this category of symptoms by using information gathered from depression or Parkinson's disease.

Conflict of interest

The authors declare no conflict of interest.

Author details

Mihaela Fadgyas Stanculete* and Octavia Capatina
Department of Neurosciences, University of Medicine and Pharmacy Iuliu Hatieganu, Cluj Napoca, Romania

*Address all correspondence to: mihaelastanculete@yahoo.com

References

[1] Kahn R, Sommer I, Murray R, Meyer-Lindenberg A, Weinberger D, Cannon T et al. Schizophrenia. Nature Reviews Disease Primers. 2015;1(1).

[2] Charlson F, Ferrari A, Santomauro D, Diminic S, Stockings E, Scott J et al. Global Epidemiology and Burden of Schizophrenia: Findings From the Global Burden of Disease Study 2016. Schizophrenia Bulletin. 2018;44(6):1195-1203.

[3] Lindenmayer, J. P., Grochowski, S., & Hyman, R. B. (1995). Five factor model of schizophrenia: replication across samples. *Schizophrenia research*, *14*(3), 229-234.

[4] Wallwork, R. S., Fortgang, R., Hashimoto, R., Weinberger, D. R., & Dickinson, D. (2012). Searching for a consensus five-factor model of the Positive and Negative Syndrome Scale for schizophrenia. *Schizophrenia research*, *137*(1-3), 246-250.

[5] van der Gaag, M., Cuijpers, A., Hoffman, T., Remijsen, M., Hijman, R., de Haan, L., ... & Wiersma, D. (2006). The five-factor model of the Positive and Negative Syndrome Scale I: confirmatory factor analysis fails to confirm 25 published five-factor solutions. *Schizophrenia research*, *85*(1-3), 273-279.

[6] Fervaha, G., Foussias, G., Agid, O., & Remington, G. (2014). Impact of primary negative symptoms on functional outcomes in schizophrenia. *European Psychiatry*, *29*(7), 449-455.

[7] Jonathan Rabinowitz, Stephen Z. Levine, George Garibaldi, Dragana Bugarski-Kirola, Carmen Galani Berardo, Shitij Kapur,Negative symptoms have greater impact on functioning than positive symptoms in schizophrenia: Analysis of CATIE data,Schizophrenia Research, Volume 137, Issues 1-3,

[8] Foussias, G., Agid, O., Fervaha, G., & Remington, G. (2014). Negative symptoms of schizophrenia: clinical features, relevance to real world functioning and specificity versus other CNS disorders. *European Neuropsychopharmacology*, *24*(5), 693-709.

[9] Correll CU, Schooler NR. Negative Symptoms in Schizophrenia: A Review and Clinical Guide for Recognition, Assessment, and Treatment. Neuropsychiatr Dis Treat. 2020 Feb 21;16:519-534. doi: 10.2147/NDT.S225643. PMID: 32110026; PMCID: PMC7041437.

[10] Harvey PD, Strassnig M. Predicting the severity of everyday functional disability in people with schizophrenia: cognitive deficits, functional capacity, symptoms, and health status. World Psychiatry. 2012;11(2):73-79. doi:10.1016/j.wpsyc.2012.05.004

[11] Foussias, G., Mann, S., Zakzanis, K. K., Van Reekum, R., Agid, O., & Remington, G. (2011). Prediction of longitudinal functional outcomes in schizophrenia: the impact of baseline motivational deficits. *Schizophrenia research*, *132*(1), 24-27.

[12] CĂPĂȚÎNĂ, O., & MICLUȚIA, I. (2018). Internalized stigma as a predictor of quality of life in schizophrenia. *Journal of Evidence-Based Psychotherapies*, *18*(2), 35-53.

[13] Sicras-Mainar, A., Maurino, J., Ruiz-Beato, E., & Navarro-Artieda, R. (2014). Impact of negative symptoms on healthcare resource utilization and associated costs in adult outpatients with schizophrenia: a population-based study. *BMC psychiatry*, *14*(1), 1-8.

[14] Möller HJ. The Relevance of Negative Symptoms in Schizophrenia and How to Treat Them with

Psychopharmaceuticals? Psychiatr Danub. 2016 Dec;28(4):435-440. PMID: 27855437.

[15] Fusar-Poli, P., Papanastasiou, E., Stahl, D., Rocchetti, M., Carpenter, W., Shergill, S., & McGuire, P. (2015). Treatments of negative symptoms in schizophrenia: meta-analysis of 168 randomized placebo-controlled trials. *Schizophrenia bulletin*, *41*(4), 892-899.

[16] Aleman A, Lincoln TM, Bruggeman R, Melle I, Arends J, Arango C, Knegtering H. Treatment of negative symptoms: Where do we stand, and where do we go? Schizophr Res. 2017 Aug;186:55-62. doi: 10.1016/j.schres.2016.05.015. Epub 2016 Jun 9. PMID: 27293137.

[17] Căpățînă, O.O., Micluția, I.V., & Fadgyas-Stănculete, M. (2021). Current perspectives in treating negative symptoms of schizophrenia: A narrative review (Review). Experimental and Therapeutic Medicine, 21, 276. https://doi.org/10.3892/etm.2021.9707

[18] Piskulic D, Addington J, Cadenhead KS, et al. Negative symptoms in individuals at clinical high risk of psychosis. Psychiatry Res. 2012;196(2-3):220-224. doi:10.1016/j.psychres.2012.02.018

[19] Velthorst E, Nieman DH, Becker HE, et al. Baseline differences in clinical symptomatology between ultra high risk subjects with and without a transition to psychosis. Schizophr Res. 2009;109(1– 3):60-65. doi:10.1016/j.schres.2009.02.002

[20] Makinen J, Miettunen J, Isohanni M, Koponen H. Negative symptoms in schizophrenia: a review. Nord J Psychiatry. 2008;62 (5):334-341. doi:10.1080/08039480801959307

[21] Galderisi, S., Mucci, A., Bitter, I., Libiger, J., Bucci, P., Fleischhacker, W. W., ... & Eufest Study Group. (2013). Persistent negative symptoms in first episode patients with schizophrenia: results from the European First Episode Schizophrenia Trial. *European Neuropsychopharmacology*, *23*(3), 196-204.

[22] Rabinowitz, J., Berardo, C. G., Bugarski-Kirola, D., & Marder, S. (2013). Association of prominent positive and prominent negative symptoms and functional health, well-being, healthcare-related quality of life and family burden: a CATIE analysis. *Schizophrenia research*, *150*(2-3), 339-342.

[23] Bobes, J., Arango, C., Garcia-Garcia, M., & Rejas, J. (2009). Prevalence of negative symptoms in outpatients with schizophrenia spectrum disorders treated with antipsychotics in routine clinical practice: findings from the CLAMORS study. *The Journal of clinical psychiatry*, *71*(3), 280-286.

[24] Austin SF, Mors O, Budtz-Jorgensen E, et al. Long-term trajectories of positive and negative symptoms in first episode psychosis: a 10year follow-up study in the OPUS cohort. Schizophr Res. 2015;168(1-2):84-91. doi:10.1016/j.schres.2015.07.021

[25] Heilbronner U, Samara M, Leucht S, Falkai P, Schulze TG. The Longitudinal Course of Schizophrenia Across the Lifespan: Clinical, Cognitive, and Neurobiological Aspects. Harv Rev Psychiatry. 2016 Mar-Apr;24(2):118-28. doi: 10.1097/HRP.0000000000000092. PMID: 26954596; PMCID: PMC5079232.

[26] Pogue-Geile MF, Harrow M. Negative symptoms in schizophrenia: their longitudinal course and prognostic importance. Schizophr Bull. 1985;11(3):427-439. doi:10.1093/schbul/11.3.427

[27] Marneros A, Andreasen N, Tsuang M. Negative versus positive

schizophrenia. Berlin: Springer-Verlag; 1991.

[28] Malaspina D, Walsh-Messinger J, Gaebel W, Smith L, Gorun A, Prudent V et al. Negative symptoms, past and present: A historical perspective and moving to DSM-5. European Neuropsychopharmacology. 2014;24(5):710-724.

[29] Kraepelin E. Dementia praecox and paraphrenia. Miami, FL: HardPress Pub.; 2013.

[30] Andreasen N. The evolving concept of schizophrenia: From Kraepelin to the present and future. Schizophrenia Research. 1997;28(2-3):105-109.

[31] Ban TA. Fifty years chlorpromazine: a historical perspective. Neuropsychiatric Disease and Treatment. 2007;3(4):495-500.

[32] Andreasen N. Negative v Positive Schizophrenia. Archives of General Psychiatry. 1982;39(7):789

[33] Crow - Crow T. The Two-syndrome Concept: Origins and Current Status. Schizophrenia Bulletin. 1985;11(3): 471-488.

[34] Carpenter W , Heinrichs D, Wagman A. Deficit and nondeficit forms of schizophrenia: the concept. American Journal of Psychiatry. 1988;145(5):578-583.

[35] Diagnostic and statistical manual of mental disorders. DSM-III-R. Prep. Washington: American Psychiatric Ass; 1987.

[36] Diagnostic and statistical manual of mental disorders. DSM-IV. Washington, DC: American Psychiatric Association; 1995.

[37] Kirkpatrick B, Buchanan R, Ross D, Carpenter W. A Separate Disease Within the Syndrome of Schizophrenia. Archives of General Psychiatry. 2001;58(2):165.

[38] Blanchard J, Horan W, Collins L. Examining the latent structure of negative symptoms: Is there a distinct subtype of negative symptom schizophrenia?. Schizophrenia Research. 2005;77(2-3):151-165.

[39] Messias E, Kirkpatrick B, Bromet E, Ross D, Buchanan B, Carpenter W et al. Summer birth and deficit schizophrenia: A pooled analysis from five countries. Schizophrenia Research. 2003; 60(1):45-46.

[40] Galderisi S, Maj M. Deficit schizophrenia: An overview of clinical, biological and treatment aspects. European Psychiatry. 2009;24(8): 493-500.

[41] Galderisi S, Quarantelli M, Volpe U, Mucci A, Cassano G, Invernizzi G et al. Patterns of Structural MRI Abnormalities in Deficit and Nondeficit Schizophrenia. Schizophrenia Bulletin. 2007;34(2):393-401.

[42] Buchanan R. Persistent Negative Symptoms in Schizophrenia: An Overview. Schizophrenia Bulletin. 2007;33(4):1013-1022.

[43] Mäkinen J, Miettunen J, Isohanni M, Koponen H. Negative symptoms in schizophrenia—A review. Nordic Journal of Psychiatry. 2008;62(5): 334-341.

[44] Kelley M, Haas G, van Kammen D. Longitudinal progression of negative symptoms in schizophrenia: A new look at an old problem. Schizophrenia Research. 2008;105(1- 3):188-196.

[45] Kirkpatrick B, Fenton W, Carpenter W, Marder S. The NIMH-MATRICS Consensus Statement on Negative Symptoms. Schizophrenia Bulletin. 2006;32(2):214-219.

[46] Blanchard J, Cohen A. The Structure of Negative Symptoms Within Schizophrenia: Implications for Assessment. Schizophrenia Bulletin. 2005;32(2):238-245.

[47] Messinger J, Trémeau F, Antonius D, Mendelsohn E, Prudent V, Stanford A et al. Avolition and expressive deficits capture negative symptom phenomenology: Implications for DSM-5 and schizophrenia research. Clinical Psychology Review. 2011;31(1):161-168.

[48] Park S, Llerena K, McCarthy J, Couture S, Bennett M, Blanchard J. Screening for negative symptoms: Preliminary results from the self-report version of the Clinical Assessment Interview for Negative Symptoms. Schizophrenia Research. 2012;135(1-3):139-143.

[49] Kirkpatrick B, Strauss G, Nguyen L, Fischer B, Daniel D, Cienfuegos A et al. The Brief Negative Symptom Scale: Psychometric Properties. Schizophrenia Bulletin. 2010;37(2):300-305. 48. Mucci A, Galderisi S. The second-generation assessment scales: Brief negative symptom scale and clinical assessment interview for negative symptoms. European Psychiatry. 2016;33:S70.

[50] Horan W, Kring A, Gur R, Reise S, Blanchard J. Development and psychometric validation of the Clinical Assessment Interview for Negative Symptoms (CAINS). Schizophrenia Research. 2011;132(2-3):140-145.

[51] Galderisi S, Bucci P, Mucci A, Kirkpatrick B, Pini S, Rossi A, Vita A, Maj M. Categorical and dimensional approaches to negative symptoms of schizophrenia: focus on long-term stability and functional outcome. Schizophr Res. 2013 Jun;147(1):157-62.

[52] Strauss GP, Horan WP, Kirkpatrick B, Fischer BA, Keller WR, Miski P, Buchanan RW, Green MF, Carpenter WT Jr. Deconstructing negative symptoms of schizophrenia: avolition-apathy and diminished expression clusters predict clinical presentation and functional outcome. J Psychiatr Res. 2013 Jun;47(6):783-90.

[53] Liemburg E, Castelein S, Stewart R, van der Gaag M, Aleman A, Knegtering H; Genetic Risk and Outcome of Psychosis (GROUP) Investigators, 2013. Two subdomains of negative symptoms in psychotic disorders: established and confirmed in two large cohorts. J. Psychiatrs. Res.47, 178-725. http://dx.doi.org/10.1016/j.jpsychires.2013.01.024

[54] Rocca P, Montemagni C, Zappia S, Piterà R, Sigaudo M, Bogetto F. Negative symptoms and everyday functioning in schizophrenia: A cross-sectional study in a real world-setting. Psychiatry Research. 2014;218(3):284-289.

[55] Galderisi S, Mucci A, Buchanan R, Arango C. Negative symptoms of schizophrenia: new developments and unanswered research questions. The Lancet Psychiatry. 2018;5(8):664-677.

[56] Marder S, Galderisi S. The current conceptualization of negative symptoms in schizophrenia. World Psychiatry. 2017;16(1):14-24.

[57] Kirkpatrick B, Castle D, Murray, R.M., Carpenter Jr WT. Risk factors for the deficit syndrome of schizophrenia. Schizophr. Bull. 2000: 26 (1), 233-242.

[58] Kirkpatrick B. The deficit syndrome: Marker of a separate disease within schizophrenia. Biological Psychiatry. 1997;42(1):203S.

[59] Turetsky BI, Colbath EA, Gur RE. P300 subcomponent abnormalities in schizophrenia: I. Physiological evidence for gender and subtype specific differences in regional pathology. Biol. Psychiatry. 1998; 43 (2), 84-96.

[60] Galderisi S, Quarantelli M, Volpe U, Mucci A, Cassano GB, Invernizzi G, Rossi A, Vita A, Pini S, Cassano P, Daneluzzo E, De Peri L, Stratta P, Brunetti A, Maj M. Patterns of structural MRI abnormalities in deficit and nondeficit schizophrenia. Schizophr. Bull.2008;34 (2), 393-401.

[61] Gonul A, Kula M, Eşel E, Tutuş A, Sofuoglu S. A Tc-99m HMPAO SPECT study of regional cerebral blood flow in drug-free schizophrenic patients with deficit and non-deficit syndrome. Psychiatry Research: Neuroimaging. 2003;123(3):199-205.

[62] Tamminga C. Limbic System Abnormalities Identified in Schizophrenia Using Positron Emission Tomography With Fluorodeoxyglucose and Neocortical Alterations With Deficit Syndrome. Archives of General Psychiatry. 1992;49(7):522-530.

[63] Mucci A, Dima D, Soricelli A, Volpe U, Bucci P, Frangou S et al. Is avolition in schizophrenia associated with a deficit of dorsal caudate activity? A functional magnetic resonance imaging study during reward anticipation and feedback. Psychological Medicine. 2015;45(08):1765-1778.

[64] Morris R, Quail S, Griffiths K, Green M, Balleine B. Corticostriatal Control of Goal-Directed Action Is Impaired in Schizophrenia. Biological Psychiatry. 2015;77(2):187-195.

[65] Lindenmayer J, Khan A, Iskander A, Abad M, Parker B. A Randomized Controlled Trial of Olanzapine Versus Haloperidol in the Treatment of Primary Negative Symptoms and Neurocognitive Deficits in Schizophrenia. The Journal of Clinical Psychiatry. 2007;68(03):368-379.

[66] Murphy B, Chung Y, Park T, McGorry P. Pharmacological treatment of primary negative symptoms in schizophrenia: A systematic review. Schizophrenia Research. 2006;88(1- 3):5-25.

[67] Leucht S. Amisulpride, an Unusual "Atypical" Antipsychotic: A Meta-Analysis of Randomized Controlled Trials. American Journal of Psychiatry. 2002;159(2):180-190.

[68] Möller H, Riedel M, Müller N, Fischer W, Kohnen R. Zotepine Versus Placebo in the Treatment of Schizophrenic Patients with Stable Primary Negative Symptoms: A Randomized Double-Blind Multicenter Trial. Pharmacopsychiatry. 2004;37(6):270-278.

[69] Maj M, Galderisi S. Deficit schizophrenia: a valid categorical subtype of schizophrenia?. Schizophrenia Research. 2008;102(1-3):45.

[70] Arango C, Garibaldi G, Marder S. Pharmacological approaches to treating negative symptoms: A review of clinical trials. Schizophrenia Research. 2013;150(2-3):346-352.

[71] Üçok A, Ergül C. Persistent negative symptoms after first episode schizophrenia: A 2-year follow-up study. Schizophrenia Research. 2014;158(1-3):241-246.

[72] López-Díaz Á, Lara I, Lahera G. Is the Prevalence of the Deficit Syndrome in Schizophrenia Higher than Estimated? Results of a Meta-Analysis. Psychiatry Investigation. 2018;15(1):94-98.

[73] Bobes J, Arango C, Garcia-Garcia M, Rejas J. Prevalence of Negative Symptoms in Outpatients With Schizophrenia Spectrum Disorders Treated With Antipsychotics in Routine Clinical Practice. The Journal of Clinical Psychiatry. 2009;71(03):280-286.

[74] Meisenzahl E, Koutsouleris N, Bottlender R, Scheuerecker J, Jäger M,

Teipel S et al. Structural brain alterations at different stages of schizophrenia: A voxel-based morphometric study. Schizophrenia Research. 2008;104(1-3):44-60.

[75] Sigmundsson T, Suckling J, Maier M, Williams S, Bullmore E, Greenwood K et al. Structural Abnormalities in Frontal, Temporal, and Limbic Regions and Interconnecting White Matter Tracts in Schizophrenic Patients With Prominent Negative Symptoms. American Journal of Psychiatry. 2001;158(2):234-243.

[76] Bodnar M, Hovington C, Buchy L, Malla A, Joober R, Lepage M. Cortical Thinning in Temporo-Parietal Junction (TPJ) in Non-Affective First-Episode of Psychosis Patients with Persistent Negative Symptoms. PLoS ONE. 2014;9(6):e101372.

[77] Hovington C, Lepage M. Neurocognition and neuroimaging of persistent negative symptoms of schizophrenia. Expert Review of Neurotherapeutics. 2012;12(1):53-69.

[78] Orsolini L, Valchera A, De Berardis D, Vecchiotti R, Iasevoli F. The novel antipsychotic cariprazine (RGH-188): State-of-the-art in the treatment of psychiatric disorders. European Psychiatry. 2016;33:S228.

[79] Nemeth G, Laszlovszky I, Czobor P, et al. Cariprazine versus risperidone monotherapy for treatment of predominant negative symptoms in patients with schizophrenia: a randomised, double-blind, controlled trial. Lancet 2017; 389: 1103-13.

[80] Davidson M, Saoud J, Staner C, Noel N, Luthringer E, Werner S et al. Efficacy and Safety of MIN-101: A 12-Week Randomized, Double-Blind, Placebo-Controlled Trial of a New Drug in Development for the Treatment of Negative Symptoms in Schizophrenia. American Journal of Psychiatry. 2017;174(12):1195-1202.

[81] Morris RW, Quail S, Griffiths KR, Green MJ, Balleine BW. Corticostriatal control of goaldirected action is impaired in schizophrenia. Biol Psychiatry 2015; 77: 187-95.

[82] Galderisi S, Färden A, Kaiser S. Dissecting negative symptoms of schizophrenia: History, assessment, pathophysiological mechanisms and treatment. Schizophrenia Research. 2017;186:1-2.

[83] Trémeau F, Nolan K, Malaspina D, Javitt D. Behavioral validation of avolition in schizophrenia. Schizophrenia Research. 2012; 138(2-3):255-261.

[84] Barch DM, Pagliaccio D, Luking K. Mechanisms underlying motivational deficits in psychopathology: similarities and differences in depression and schizophrenia. Curr Topics Behav Neurosci 2016; 27: 411-49.

[85] Radua J, Schmidt A, Borgwardt S, et al. Ventral striatal activation during reward processing in psychosis: a neurofunctional meta-analysis. JAMA Psychiatry 2015; 72: 1243-51.

[86] Beck A, Grant P, Huh G, Perivoliotis D, Chang N. Dysfunctional Attitudes and Expectancies in Deficit Syndrome Schizophrenia. Schizophrenia Bulletin. 2011; 39(1):43-51.

[87] Grant P. Randomized Trial to Evaluate the Efficacy of Cognitive Therapy for LowFunctioning Patients With Schizophrenia. Archives of General Psychiatry. 2012;69(2):121-127.

[88] Lindenmayer J, Nasrallah H, Pucci M, James S, Citrome L. A systematic review of psychostimulant treatment of negative symptoms of schizophrenia: Challenges and therapeutic opportunities. Schizophrenia Research. 2013;147(2-3):241-252.

[89] Sethom M, Fares S, Bouaziz N, Melki W, Jemaa R, Feki M et al. Polyunsaturated fatty acids deficits are associated with psychotic state and negative symptoms in patients with schizophrenia. Prostaglandins, Leukotrienes and Essential Fatty Acids. 2010;83(3):131- 136.

[90] Tsapakis E, Dimopoulou T, Tarazi F. Clinical management of negative symptoms of schizophrenia: An update. Pharmacology & Therapeutics. 2015;153:135-147.

[91] Ellman L, Cook A, Schaefer C, Bresnahan M, Susser E, Brown A. 113. Maternal inflammation during pregnancy and symptom profiles of offspring diagnosed with schizophrenia. Brain, Behavior, and Immunity. 2014;40:e33.

[92] Oya K, Kishi T, Iwata N. Efficacy and tolerability of minocycline augmentation therapy in schizophrenia: a systematic review and meta-analysis of randomized controlled trials. Human Psychopharmacology: Clinical and Experimental. 2014;29(5):483-491.

[93] Freitas C, Fregni F, Pascual-Leone A. Meta-analysis of the effects of repetitive transcranial magnetic stimulation (rTMS) on negative and positive symptoms in schizophrenia. Schizophrenia Research. 2009;108(1-3):11-24.

[94] Dlabač-de Lange J, Knegtering R, Aleman A. Repetitive Transcranial Magnetic Stimulation for Negative Symptoms of Schizophrenia. The Journal of Clinical Psychiatry. 2010;71(04):411-418.

[95] Smith R, Boules S, Mattiuz S, Youssef M, Tobe R, Sershen H et al. Effects of transcranial direct current stimulation (tDCS) on cognition, symptoms, and smoking in schizophrenia: A randomized controlled study. Schizophrenia Research. 2015;168(1-2):260-266.

[96] Fitzgerald P, McQueen S, Daskalakis Z, Hoy K. A Negative Pilot Study of Daily Bimodal Transcranial Direct Current Stimulation in Schizophrenia. Brain Stimulation. 2014;7(6):813-816.

[97] Cohen A, Morrison S, Brown L, Minor K. Towards a cognitive resource limitations model of diminished expression in schizotypy. Journal of Abnormal Psychology. 2012;121(1):109-118.

[98] Lepage M, Sergerie K, Benoit A, Czechowska Y, Dickie E, Armony J. Emotional face processing and flat affect in schizophrenia: functional and structural neural correlates. Psychological Medicine. 2011;41(09): 1833-1844.

[99] Stip E, Fahim C, Liddle P, Mancini-Marïe A, Mensour B, Bentaleb L et al. Neural Correlates of Sad Feelings in Schizophrenia with and without Blunted Affect. The Canadian Journal of Psychiatry. 2005;50(14):909-917.

[100] Aleman A, Kahn R. Strange feelings: do amygdala abnormalities dysregulate the emotional brain in schizophrenia? Prog. Neurobiol. 2005;77 (5), 283-298.

[101] Hager O, Kirschner, M, Bischof M, Hartmann-Riemer M, Kluge A, Seifritz E, Tobler P, Kaiser S. Reward-dependent modulation of working memory is associated with negative symptoms in schizophrenia. Schizophr. Res. 2015;168 (1-2), 238-244.

[102] Bor J, Brunelin J, d'Amato T, Costes N, Suaud-Chagny M, Saoud M et al. How can cognitive remediation therapy modulate brain activations in schizophrenia?. Psychiatry Research: Neuroimaging. 2011;192(3):160-166.

[103] Elis O, Caponigro J, Kring A. Psychosocial treatments for negative symptoms in schizophrenia: Current practices and future directions. Clinical Psychology Review. 2013;33(8):914-928.

[104] De Berardis D, Marini S, Iasevoli F, Tomasetti C, deBartolomeis A, Mazza M, Valchera A. The role of intranasaloxytocinin the treatment of patients with schizophrenia: a systematic review. CNSNeurol. Disord. DrugTargets. 2013:12:252-264.

[105] Sullivan PF, Kendler KS, Neale MC. Schizophrenia as a complex trait: evidence from a meta-analysis of twin studies. Archives of general psychiatry. 2003 Dec 1;60(12):1187-92.

[106] Fanous AH, Van Den Oord EJ, Riley BP, Aggen SH, Neale MC, O'neill FA, Walsh D, Kendler KS. Relationship between a high-risk haplotype in the DTNBP1 (dysbindin) gene and clinical features of schizophrenia. American Journal of Psychiatry. 2005 Oct 1;162(10):1824-32.

[107] DeRosse P, Funke B, Burdick KE, Lencz T, Ekholm JM, Kane JM, Kucherlapati R, Malhotra AK. Dysbindin genotype and negative symptoms in schizophrenia. American Journal of Psychiatry. 2006 Mar 1;163(3):532-4.

[108] Pelayo-Terán JM, Crespo-Facorro B, Carrasco-Marín E, Pérez-Iglesias R, Mata I, Arranz MJ, Leyva-Cobián F, Vázquez-Barquero JL. Catechol-O-methyltransferase Val158Met polymorphism and clinical characteristics in first episode non-affective psychosis. American Journal of Medical Genetics Part B: Neuropsychiatric Genetics. 2008 Jul 5;147(5):550-6.

[109] Wessman J, Paunio T, Tuulio-Henriksson A, Koivisto M, Partonen T, Suvisaari J, Turunen JA, Wedenoja J, Hennah W, Pietiläinen OP, Lönnqvist J. Mixture model clustering of phenotype features reveals evidence for association of DTNBP1 to a specific subtype of schizophrenia. Biological psychiatry. 2009 Dec 1;66(11):990-6.

[110] Bertolino A, Fazio L, Caforio G, Blasi G, Rampino A, Romano R, Di Giorgio A, Taurisano P, Papp A, Pinsonneault J, Wang D. Functional variants of the dopamine receptor D2 gene modulate prefronto-striatal phenotypes in schizophrenia. Brain. 2009 Feb 1;132(2):417-25.

[111] Petrovsky N, Quednow BB, Ettinger U, Schmechtig A, Mössner R, Collier DA, Kühn KU, Maier W, Wagner M, Kumari V. Sensorimotor gating is associated with CHRNA3 polymorphisms in schizophrenia and healthy volunteers. Neuropsychopharmacology. 2010 Jun;35(7):1429-39.

[112] Xu C, Aragam N, Li X, Villla EC, Wang L, Briones D, Petty L, Posada Y, Arana TB, Cruz G, Mao C. BCL9 and C9orf5 are associated with negative symptoms in schizophrenia: meta-analysis of two genome-wide association studies. PloS one. 2013 Jan 29;8(1):e51674.

[113] Mezquida G, Penades R, Cabrera B, Savulich G, Lobo A, González-Pinto A, Penzol MJ, Corripio I, Fernandez-Egea E, Gassó P, Cuesta MJ. Association of the brain-derived neurotrophic factor Val66Met polymorphism with negative symptoms severity, but not cognitive function, in first-episode schizophrenia spectrum disorders. European Psychiatry. 2016 Oct;38:61-9.

[114] Edwards AC, Bigdeli TB, Docherty AR, Bacanu S, Lee D, De Candia TR, Moscati A, Thiselton DL, Maher BS, Wormley BK, Molecular Genetics of Schizophrenia Collaboration (MGS). Meta-analysis of positive and negative symptoms reveals

schizophrenia modifier genes. Schizophrenia bulletin. 2016 Mar 1;42(2):279-87.

[115] Gao J, Yi H, Tang X, Feng X, Yu M, Sha W, Wang X, Zhang X, Zhang X. DNA methylation and gene expression of matrix metalloproteinase 9 gene in deficit and non-deficit schizophrenia. Frontiers in genetics. 2018 Dec 11;9:646.

[116] Schneider M, Armando M, Schultze-Lutter F, Pontillo M, Vicari S, Debbané M, Eliez S. Prevalence, course and psychosis-predictive value of negative symptoms in 22q11. 2 deletion syndrome. Schizophrenia research. 2019 Apr 1;206:386-93.

Section 3

Pathophysiology

Chapter 5

Role of Immunity in Pathogenesis of Psychosis

Wafa Abdelghaffar, Oussama Sidhom, Lilia Laadhar and Rym Rafrafi

Abstract

The involvement of immunity in the pathogenesis of schizophrenia and related psychoses was suspected a century ago but was shadowed by the dopaminergic hypothesis after the discovery of antipsychotics. We currently know that this latter theory has many limits and cannot account for the wide variety of psychotic conditions. The immune-inflammatory theory is now one of the most promising axes of research in terms of pathogenesis of several mental health conditions. Immunity and inflammation play a role at least in a subgroup of patients with psychosis. The immune system is complex with a variety of components and mediators that can all have effects on the brain and thus mediate psychiatric symptoms. In this chapter we will explore the scientific evidence of the role of immune system in pathophysiology of psychosis. The sections of this chapter will discuss the role of innate system components (cytokines, microglia, inflammation.), the role of adaptive system (lymphocytes and antibodies) with a section focusing on auto-immunity and particularly antineuronal antibodies. Finally we will discuss how this research can impact patients management and elaborate recommendations for future research.

Keywords: schizophrenia, psychosis, inflammation, auto-immunity, antineuronal antibodies, pathophysiology

1. Introduction

The role of the immune system in mental disorders was suspected since the last century [1]. Then, the discovery of efficient antipsychotic drugs led researches to focus on the dopaminergic theory undermining the first immunological findings. Nonetheless, this theory has many limits and cannot account for the wide diversity of clinical presentations in patients with psychosis. In the last decades, there was a breakthrough in technical investigations that led to significant improvement of our understanding of the immune system functioning and the immune theory became a promising axis of research.

The immune system has a complex organization with an innate system (mediated by macrophages, neutrophils and cytokines) and an adaptive system which is antigen specific (mediated by T and B lymphocytes and antibodies secreted by B lymphocytes).

Many researchers have found immunological abnormalities in patients with psychosis involving both the innate and the adaptive system [2]. All immune system components can have effects on the brain cells and thus they can produce psychiatric symptoms [2]. Increase in inflammation markers was detected in schizophrenia [3]. Early life and prenatal exposition to infections predicted adult schizophrenia [4, 5]. High rates of auto-antibodies were reported in psychiatric conditions especially antineuronal antibodies [6–8]. There are genetic findings that also consolidate these theories [9]. All these findings allow to conclude that immunity plays a role in pathophysiology of psychosis at least in a subgroup of patients. There are already trials using treatments targeting the immune system with encouraging results [10]. This axis of research can have an impact on the understanding and treatment of schizophrenia and related psychoses and allow a new era of immuno-psychiatry.

2. Evidence of involvement of immune system in pathogenesis of psychosis

2.1 Role of inflammation and innate immune system

Inflammation and innate system are the first line response, nonspecific to an antigen, when an infection occurs. It involves neutrophils, macrophages, microglia and secretion of acute-phase proteins like inflammatory cytokines. There is evidence for inflammation dysfunction in psychosis. Interleukins and C Reactive Protein (CRP) increase in patients with psychosis [11, 12]. An increase in the production of proinflammatory cytokines such as Interleukin 6 (IL-6) was detected in patients with schizophrenia [13] and patients at high risk for psychosis [14] and predicted development of adult schizophrenia when detected in children [4]. This increase in IL-6 was also found in the cerebrospinal fluid [15] in schizophrenia patients. A meta-analysis showed that pro-inflammatory cytokines increased in acute psychosis phase either during a first episode or during a relapse, and normalized after antipsychotic treatment [16]. Thus, these markers could be used to detect acute psychosis and predict relapses. Peripheral inflammation can also affect the brain [17]. In fact, inflammation can activate endothelial cells in brain vessels and increase their permeability to immunological cells [18]. Moreover, inflammation that begins in periphery can reach the brain, probably through vagus nerve signals [17] and can activate microglia. Microglia is an essential component of central nervous system and has a hemopoietic origin [19]. Inflammation can activate microglia which in turn can release cytokines in the brain. Microglia also interacts with lymphocytes and can play a role of antigen presenting cell. This is consistent with the "microglia activation hypothesis" [20] that emphasizes the role of cytokines and free radicals produced by the activated microglia in pathophysiology of psychosis. Those substances can cause white matter and neurogenesis abnormalities and neuronal alterations associated with psychosis. Cytokines can also amplify the oxidative stress via toxic nitric oxide, which in turn, activates the hypothalamic–pituitary–adrenal axis [17]. This leads to the activation of the corticosteroid system that releases stress hormones such as cortisol [17, 21]. All these inflammatory processes could result in mood and cognition disturbances in humans [18, 22] through direct effect on the brain and through the cortisol secretion alterations. Corticosteroid levels alterations are known to induce affective and behavioral disturbances.
The activation of corticosteroid system by cytokines following an inflammatory immune response has already been demonstrated in major depressive disorder and could also be part of the pathophysiology of psychosis [17, 18, 22].

Schizophrenia has been associated with prenatal infections [5] and with childhood central nervous system infections [4]. These findings suggest a common underlying pathway between schizophrenia and infectious conditions involving mainly inflammatory immune response [21].

2.2 Role of lymphocytes and adaptive system

The adaptive system represents the second line antigen-specific immune response. It involves lymphocytes B and T and antibodies secreted by lymphocytes B. It also allows to keep a memory of past infections.

Findings from experimental studies found abnormalities in lymphocytes function and number in patients with schizophrenia, particularly T-cells [12, 22]. Interleukin 2 (Il-2) is involved in immune response regulation. T cells of schizophrenia patients produce reduced amounts of Il-2 in vitro [23], and schizophrenia was associated with more activated lymphocytes, expressing CD56, compared to controls [24], especially in acute relapses, with changes in the ratio CD8/CD4 cells [22]. Baseline lymphopenia can be associated with severe psychosis and predict poor outcome and poor treatment response [25]. These findings are consistent with The "macrophage-T-lymphocyte theory" postulating that cytokines produced by activated lymphocytes T and macrophages play a main role in pathophysiology of schizophrenia [26]. In fact, CD4 T-lymphocytes secrete cytokines such as IFN-γ and IL-12 which can activate CD56-lymphocytes that secrete TNF-α and IFN-γ. Pro-inflammatory cytokines are associated with schizophrenia as was shown in the previous section [16]. A decrease in CD19 B-lymphocytes count was demonstrated in patients treated with adjunctive celecoxib [27] and this was associated with negative symptoms improvement. Post-mortem studies reported evidence of microglia activation [28, 29] and increased number of lymphocytes [30] in schizophrenia. Most studies focused on blood cells count [22], while there can also be changes in cerebrospinal fluid as demonstrated by many authors [24, 31, 32].

2.3 Role of auto-immunity and antineuronal antibodies

The involvement of autoimmunity in psychosis was suspected about a century ago [1, 33]. There is evidence for the role of auto-immune antibodies, in the pathogenesis of psychiatric disorders in general and in psychosis in particular [7, 33]. Psychotic and auto-immune conditions share many clinical and biological features like a young age onset [1, 34, 35], stress-triggered [6, 36], they have chronic course with relapses and possible residual symptoms [6, 34]. Besides, psychosis is often associated with auto-immune conditions [35] and high levels of auto-immune antibodies were found in patients with psychosis (e.g. antibodies anti-gliadin and anti-casein) [7, 37] and particularly antineuronal antibodies [2, 8, 38]. Antineuronal antibodies can target cell surface components, such as the N-Methyl D Aspartate (NMDA) receptor, or they can target intra-cellular nuclear or cytoplasmic antigens.

The most studied antineuronal antibodies in the literature are cell surface antibodies anti-NMDA [38]. Patients with anti-NMDA antibodies often present with predominant psychotic symptoms and subsequently develop other neurological symptoms [39]. This is called NMDA encephalitis and can be treated using immunotherapy and removal of auto-antibodies [40]. Some patients have anti-NMDA and mild psychotic symptoms but have no neurological symptoms of encephalitis. Authors have suggested the concept of " auto-immune psychosis " [41, 42] to describe this entity.

There are many arguments for NMDA receptor hypofunction in schizophrenia [2, 38]. The administration of ketamine and phencyclidine, which are NMDA receptor blockers, is known to cause clinical [43, 44] and physiological symptoms [45] similar to schizophrenia. Glutamate and glycine are necessary for NMDA receptor activation and they have decreased levels in schizophrenia [38, 46, 47]. Psychosis is also associated with abnormal D-amino acids levels (including D-serine and D-alanine) [48, 49] which are modulators of neuronal activity [50] and act as co-agonists of NMDA receptor at the Glycine Modulatory Site [38, 46]. There is also an increase in antagonist agents of NMDA receptor in schizophrenia [51]. These findings were used in developing treatment trials for psychosis by augmenting NMDA receptor function [38, 41].

Antineuronal antibodies can also target intracellular antigens such as Antineuronal Nuclear Autoantibodies (ANNA) (called anti-Hu and anti-Ri) and Anti cytoplasm of Purkinje cells Antibodies (PCA) (called anti-Yo). Those antibodies have been classically associated with paraneoplastic syndromes [52, 53] but they were also found in persons with neurological or psychiatric conditions with no associated tumor [8]. For example, these antibodies were found in association with neurological diseases [54], with auto-immune diseases [55], with neuropsychiatry symptoms of neurolupus [56], with autism [57, 58] and with obsessive compulsive disorder [59, 60]. A study found ANNA antibodies were significantly higher in schizophrenia and bipolar disorder patients compared to healthy controls [8] with no tumor detected after 5 years follow up. In this study, PCA antibodies were associated with the presence of affective symptoms. Most authors are now focusing on anti-NMDA antibodies but future studies should address these antinuclear and cytoplasmic antibodies.

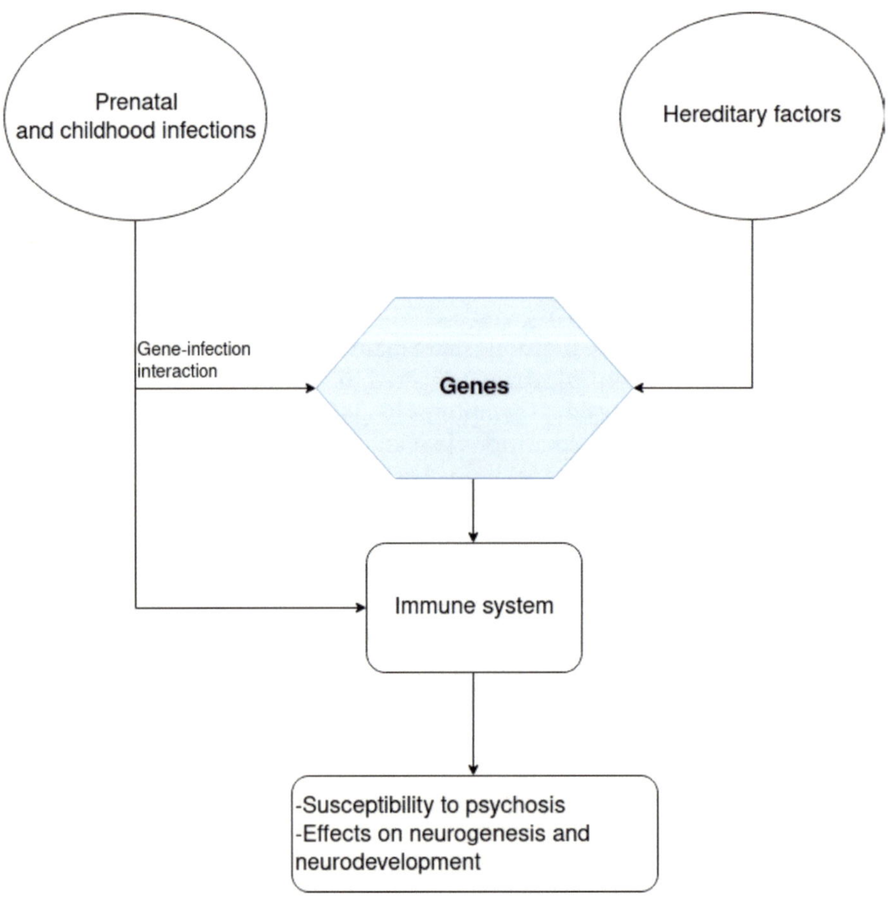

Figure 1.
Early life interactions resulting in susceptibility to psychosis.

2.4 Genetic findings

Genome Wide Association Studies (GWAS) found an association between schizophrenia and genes that are related to immune system cells [61]. Another GWAS showed that a single nucleotide polymorphism in major histocompatibility complex on chromosome 6 was associated with schizophrenia [62]. This region of chromosome 6 includes genes expressing proteins involved in pro-inflammatory cytokines. A genetic association was also found between schizophrenia and multiple sclerosis, an immune mediated disease [63].

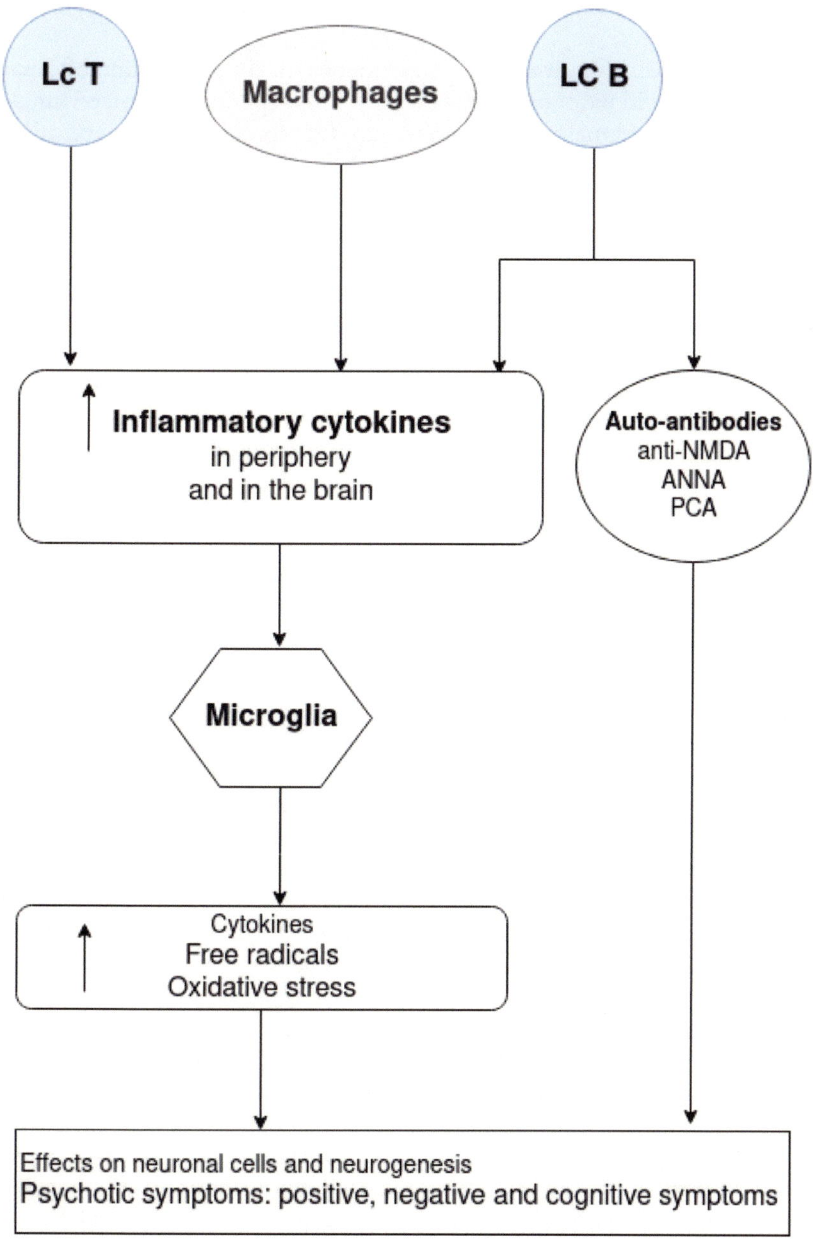

Figure 2.
Simplified diagram of possible immune interactions resulting in psychotic symptoms. Lc, lymphocyte; NMDA, N-methyl D-aspartate receptor; ANNA, antinuclear neuronal antibodies; PCA, anti Purkinje cell cytoplasm antibodies.

As we previously discussed, NMDA-receptor downregulation is associated with schizophrenia. A meta-analysis showed that there is hypoexpression of the mRNA of a subunit of NMDA receptor called GluN1 [64] in schizophrenia. Besides, the expression and activity of DAAO, an enzyme that catabolizes D-amino acids which act like agonists of NMDA receptor, are increased and DAAO gene is considered as risk gene for schizophrenia [65].

During the early life and prenatal development, the association between genetic susceptibility and early infections can affect immunological pathways illustrating the gene-infection interaction (**Figure 1**).

2.5 Summary of immune systems interactions leading to psychotic symptoms

In the previous sections, we presented evidence for the implication of innate and adaptive system in psychosis pathogenesis. This separation between innate and adaptive systems is schematic and is usually used for its clarity. In reality, all these components interact with each other in order to perform an adequate immunological response to infection (**Figure 2**). How do all these systems interact and lead to psychosis symptoms? In a classic immune response to an infection, innate system is the first actor through macrophages activation and cytokines secretion. Then, T and B-lymphocytes are activated and also produce inflammatory cytokines. On the one hand, inflammation activates microglia in the brain which in turn secretes inflammatory cytokines. This environment of inflammation and oxidative stress could lead to hypothalamic activation and then corticosteroid system activation with release of stress hormones. Oxidative stress within the brain and stress hormones are known to account for mood and behavioral disturbances. On the other hand, B-lymphocytes can secrete auto-antibodies that react with neuronal brain cells. These antineuronal antibodies can target cell surface (such as anti-NMDA) or target intracellular antigens (such as ANNA and PCA). All these auto-antibodies were associated in the literature with psychiatric conditions.

3. Treatment implications

Antipsychotics, either first or second generation, were the only treatments used in patients with psychosis for decades. Nonetheless, they have many limitations. They are quite effective on positive symptoms but they failed at treating negative and cognitive dimensions or global functioning [66]. Moreover, there is a significant rate of treatment resistance of nearly 30% [67]. Besides, they can induce severe neurological, metabolic or hematologic side effects [68]. The rationale of these treatments is based on the dopaminergic theory which cannot account for all aspects and symptoms of psychosis. Thus, researchers are looking for treatment alternatives.

Given the substancial evidence of immune dysfunction in psychosis, scientists have tried medications acting on the immune system. There have been many trials with anti-inflammatory medications combined with antipsychotics [10] using aspirin [69, 70], celecoxib [27, 71, 72] and N-acetyl-Cystein [73, 74] with encouraging results (**Table 1**). Celecoxib [27] and N-acetylcysteine [73, 74] were associated with negative symptoms improvement. Meta-analyses about adjunctive minocycline, a tetracycline antibiotic with anti-inflammatory properties, found global improvement in PANSS total score [76] and cognitive function [77, 80]. Two meta-analyses assessed trials using other molecules with anti-inflammatory and neuroprotective properties such as eicosapentaenoic acid, pregnonolone, estrogens, Selective Estrogen Receptor Modulators [77] and statins [79]. Only eicosapentaenoic acid

Adjunctive therapy	Main trials results
N-Acetyl-Cystein	PANSS improv [73]; Neg symp improv [74];
Aspirin	PANSS improv [69, 70]
Celecoxib	PANSS improv [71, 75]; Neg symp improv [27]; No signif improv [72]
Minocycline	PANSS improv [76]
Pregnenolone	PANSS improv, Cognitive improv (5 trials) [77]
Estrogen	PANSS improv (8 trials) [77]
Erythropoietin	Cognitive improv [78]
Eicosapentaenoic acid	No sig improv (20 trials) [77]
Statins	PANSS improv [79] with negative symp improv on simvastatine
Tocilizimab	Negative symptoms improv [80]; no signif improv [81]
NMDA modulators	No cog improv [82, 83]; negative symptoms improv in UHR [84]

improv, improvement; no signif, no significant; PANSS improv, PANSS total score improvement; UHR, Ultra High Risk for psychosis.

Table 1.
Main results of trials using adjunctive immunotherapy combined with antipsychotics.

was not associated with significant clinical improvement. Results reported global improvement in total PANNSS scores on all other agents and cognitive function improvement on pregnonolone and negative symptoms improvement on simvastatine. A pilot trial demonstrated improvement of cognitive function on recombinant human erythropoietin [78]. Despite limitations, like study sample size, and despite the presence of some negative results [70, 72], authors reported promising results. There was an overall good tolerance.

Some biological agents can act as inflammatory response modulators, such as monoclonal antibodies and mesenchymal stem cells, and were studied in recent trials in neurological and psychiatric disorders like autism and schizophrenia [85]. Trials using adjunctive monoclonal antibodies, like tocilizumab and canakinumab, in psychosis reported improvement in negative [80] or positive symptoms [86] or no significant improvement [81].

There is another axis of research based on NMDA receptor augmenting strategies based on the increase of agonists of this receptor or decrease of antagonists. There were tens of placebo controlled trials using agonists of Glycerine Modulatory Site in NMDA receptor [38] such as glycine or D-amino acids. The results were mixed [38, 82]. Methodological bias and differences in the used molecules can account for the variability of the results. A meta-analysis did not find improvement in cognitive function using glutamate positive modulators in schizophrenia [83]. However a pilot study showed an improvement in negative symptoms using D-serine, which is an agonist of NMDA receptor, in teenagers with high risk of psychosis [84]. Thus, it could be useful to use NMDA augmenting in prevention for early psychosis stages (**Table 1**).

Clinical trials are now focusing on anti-inflammatory strategies and NMDA augmenting. It would be useful to widen our perspective and consider other therapeutic options. For example, we could consider treatments inspired from well-established auto-immune conditions like removal of antibodies or immunosuppression. Many of the trials mentioned above still suffer from lack of data. There are limitations to the generalization and clinical application of these therapies. There are confounding factors like the type of antipsychotic drug used in combination, patients compliance, inclusion criteria, illness stage, medical history and other factors that modulate immune response such as body mass, smoking status, or associated stress. All these factors need to be addressed and controlled in larger studies. However, despite these limitations, we can notice that there is accumulative evidence of the potential of anti-inflammatory and immunotherapy strategies in treating patients with psychosis. We need a better definition of patients subgroups and specific symptoms that could benefit from these therapies. A stratification of patients could be made using the immunological status and/or clinical dimensions.

4. Recommendations for future research

It is now clear that we should not limit our research and treatment strategies to antipsychotics. Immunological alterations seem to account for psychotic symptoms in a subgroup of patients. These patients can benefit from immunotherapy. The challenge is to better characterize this subgroup and define the features that predict a good response to immunotherapy. A stratification should be made using biological markers, clinical symptoms, response to antipsychotic treatments, disease stage etc. We could define an immune phenotype that predicts treatment response. It was used successfully in a trial about depression [87]. In this trial, patients who had baseline high levels of inflammatory mediators had significant improvement of depressive symptoms on infliximab which is an anti-inflammatory agent. This approach should be explored in psychosis.

Some clinical symptoms do not respond well to antipsychotics like the negative and cognitive dimensions [66]. These symptoms could benefit from other therapeutic strategies. As mentioned above, many immunotherapy trials reported improvement in negative or cognitive domains [27, 74, 76, 78, 79]. There are arguments that corroborate this theory: inflammation was associated with impairments in memory and learning [88] and in spatial memory [89]. There is still no established physiopathology accounting for immune therapies effects on negative and cognitive symptoms but hypothetical mechanisms can be proposed. Inflammation and cytokines are associated with cognitive impairments [88, 89]. Inflammation is also incriminated in the genesis of negative symptoms and motivational deficits through the action of cytokines on basal ganglia and through decrease of neuronal activity in reward system [90]. Thus, anti-inflammatory drugs could improve cognitive symptoms by reducing inflammation.

All these clinical and biological features (i.e. negative and cognitive symptoms, inflammatory phenotype etc.) should be considered as endophenotypes related to psychosis and used to categorize and stratify patients in future trials. A subgroup of patients with schizophrenia could have immune alterations accounting for psychotic symptoms and would be more prone to respond to immune therapy. This subgroup could have some characteristics: prominent negative symptoms and cognitive dysfunction, poor response to conventional treatments, a specific immune phenotype characterized for example by elevated baseline inflammatory markers or increased lymphocytes number. The immune phenotype predicting therapeutic response has to be better specified in future studies (which markers? What are the specific sub-types of lymphocytes? Etc). The duration of illness can influence clinical presentation and treatment response. Some immunotherapies proved more effective when administered at an early stage of psychosis [84]. A staging of psychotic conditions should be considered, as for staging used in cancers, in some immune diseases, and bipolar disorder [91].

Antipsychotic treatment resistance is a challenge for scientists and causes disability and high personal and social burden. Those patients could benefit from new generation treatments like immunotherapy. Some immunological markers can predict severe psychosis and poor treatment response on antipsychotics [14, 22, 25]. In the future, we could define precise immunological markers that may predict antipsychotic resistance and good response to immunotherapy.

The inflammatory status can differ between acute exacerbation phases and residual phases [16, 30]. Thus, inflammation markers could be used to predict and diagnose psychotic relapses or first episode psychoses in addition to clinical examination.

Multicenter large trials are needed with study of lymphocytes numbers and subtypes, cytokines types and with control of confounding factors. Dosage of anti-inflammatory treatments and interactions with antipsychotics should also be addressed. New strategies based on auto-immune model can broaden the therapeutic arsenal.

A novel axis of research based on the "gut-brain theory" should be considered in future research. In this theory, the intestinal microbiota composition could play a role in many central nervous system diseases through a bidirectional pathway between gut and brain [92]. Mechanisms of this interplay probably involves neurohumoral communication, vagus nerve signals and tryptophan metabolism [75].

5. Conclusions

The role of immunity in the pathogenesis of psychosis is now established, at least in a subgroup of patients. The challenge is to determine solid criteria to recognize this subgroup with possible benefit from immunotherapy. Another challenge is to develop efficient therapies based on immune system interactions with acceptable tolerance.

Conflict of interest

Authors have no conflicts of interest.

Author details

Wafa Abdelghaffar[1,3]*, Oussama Sidhom[2,4], Lilia Laadhar[1,5] and Rym Rafrafi[1,3]

1 University of Tunis El Manar, Tunisia

2 McGill University, Canada

3 Mental Health Department, Mongi Slim University Hospital, Marsa, Tunisia

4 Integrated Centre of Health and Social Services in Outaouais, Quebec, Canada

5 Immunology Department, Rabta University Hospital, Tunis, Tunisia

*Address all correspondence to: wafa.abdelghaffar@fmt.utm.tn

References

[1] Ader R. On the development of psychoneuroimmunology. In: European Journal of Pharmacology. 2000.

[2] Khandaker GM, Cousins L, Deakin J, Lennox BR, Yolken R, Jones PB. Inflammation and immunity in schizophrenia: Implications for pathophysiology and treatment. The Lancet Psychiatry. 2015.

[3] Müller N. Inflammation in schizophrenia: Pathogenetic aspects and therapeutic considerations. Schizophr Bull. 2018;

[4] Khandaker GM, Zimbron J, Dalman C, Lewis G, Jones PB. Childhood infection and adult schizophrenia: A meta-analysis of population-based studies. Schizophr Res. 2012;

[5] Khandaker GM, Zimbron J, Lewis G, Jones PB. Prenatal maternal infection, neurodevelopment and adult schizophrenia: A systematic review of population-based studies. Psychol Med. 2013;

[6] Rothermundt M, Arolt V, Bayer TA. Review of immunological and immunopathological findings in schizophrenia. Brain Behav Immun. 2001;

[7] Sidhom O, Laadhar L, Zitouni M, Ben Alaya N, Rafrafi R, Kallel-Sellami M, et al. Spectrum of autoantibodies in tunisian psychiatric inpatients. Immunol Invest. 2012 Jul;41(5):538-549.

[8] Laadhar L, Sidhom O, Sassi N, Abdelghaffar W, Lahmar H, Kallel-Sellami M, et al. High Prevalence of Antineuronal Antibodies in Tunisian Psychiatric Inpatients. J Neuropsychiatry Clin Neurosci [Internet]. 2015 [cited 2020 Dec 11];27(1):54-58. Available from: https://neuro.psychiatryonline.org/doi/abs/10.1176/appi.neuropsych.13070153

[9] Stefansson H, Ophoff RA, Steinberg S, Andreassen OA, Cichon S, Rujescu D, et al. Common variants conferring risk of schizophrenia. Nature. 2009;

[10] Hong J, Bang M. Anti-inflammatory Strategies for Schizophrenia: A review of evidence for therapeutic applications and drug repurposing. Clinical Psychopharmacology and Neuroscience. 2020.

[11] Wium-Andersen MK, Ørsted DD, Nordestgaard BG. Elevated C-reactive protein associated with late-and very-late-onset schizophrenia in the general population: A prospective study. Schizophr Bull. 2014;

[12] Wafa Abdelghaffar, Rabaa Jomli, Yosra Zgueb, Uta Ouali FN. Lymphocytes count and C-reactive protein level in patients with bipolar disorder. In: International Review of Psychosis & Bipolarity. Athen; 2014.

[13] Potvin S, Stip E, Sepehry AA, Gendron A, Bah R, Kouassi E. Inflammatory Cytokine Alterations in Schizophrenia: A Systematic Quantitative Review. Biol Psychiatry. 2008;

[14] Stojanovic A, Martorell L, Montalvo I, Ortega L, Monseny R, Vilella E, et al. Increased serum interleukin-6 levels in early stages of psychosis: Associations with at-risk mental states and the severity of psychotic symptoms. Psychoneuroendo crinology. 2014;

[15] Garver DL, Tamas RL, Holcomb JA. Elevated interleukin-6 in the cerebrospinal fluid of a previously delineated schizophrenia subtype. Neuropsychopharmacology. 2003;

[16] Miller BJ, Buckley P, Seabolt W, Mellor A, Kirkpatrick B. Meta-analysis of cytokine alterations in schizophrenia: Clinical status and antipsychotic effects. Biol Psychiatry. 2011;

[17] Dantzer R, O'Connor JC, Freund GG, Johnson RW, Kelley KW. From inflammation to sickness and depression: When the immune system subjugates the brain. Nature Reviews Neuroscience. 2008.

[18] Dantzer R. Cytokine-induced sickness behaviour: A neuroimmune response to activation of innate immunity. European Journal of Pharmacology. 2004.

[19] Hanisch UK, Kettenmann H. Microglia: Active sensor and versatile effector cells in the normal and pathologic brain. Nature Neuroscience. 2007.

[20] Monji A, Kato T, Kanba S. Cytokines and schizophrenia: Microglia hypothesis of schizophrenia. Psychiatry Clin Neurosci. 2009;

[21] Miller AH, Maletic V, Raison CL. Inflammation and Its Discontents: The Role of Cytokines in the Pathophysiology of Major Depression. Biological Psychiatry. 2009.

[22] Miller BJ, Gassama B, Sebastian D, Buckley P, Mellor A. Meta-analysis of lymphocytes in schizophrenia: Clinical status and antipsychotic effects. Biol Psychiatry. 2013;

[23] Ganguli R, Rabin BS, Kelly RH, Lyte M, Ragu U. Clinical and Laboratory Evidence of Autoimmunity in Acute Schizophrenia. Ann N Y Acad Sci. 1987;

[24] Nikkilä H V., Müller K, Ahokas A, Rimón R, Andersson LC. Increased frequency of activated lymphocytes in the cerebrospinal fluid of patients with acute schizophrenia. Schizophr Res. 2001;

[25] Zorrilla EP, Cannon TD, Kessler J, Gur RE. Leukocyte differentials predict short-term clinical outcome following antipsychotic treatment in schizophrenia. Biol Psychiatry. 1998;

[26] Smith RS, Maes M. The macrophage-T-lymphocyte theory of schizophrenia: Additional evidence. Med Hypotheses. 1995;

[27] Müller N, Krause D, Dehning S, Musil R, Schennach-Wolff R, Obermeier M, et al. Celecoxib treatment in an early stage of schizophrenia: Results of a randomized, double-blind, placebo-controlled trial of celecoxib augmentation of amisulpride treatment. Schizophr Res. 2010;

[28] Steiner J, Mawrin C, Ziegeler A, Bielau H, Ullrich O, Bernstein HG, et al. Distribution of HLA-DR-positive microglia in schizophrenia reflects impaired cerebral lateralization. Acta Neuropathol. 2006;

[29] Steiner J, Bielau H, Brisch R, Danos P, Ullrich O, Mawrin C, et al. Immunological aspects in the neurobiology of suicide: Elevated microglial density in schizophrenia and depression is associated with suicide. J Psychiatr Res. 2008;

[30] Busse S, Busse M, Schiltz K, Bielau H, Gos T, Brisch R, et al. Different distribution patterns of lymphocytes and microglia in the hippocampus of patients with residual versus paranoid schizophrenia: Further evidence for disease course-related immune alterations? Brain Behav Immun. 2012;

[31] Nikkilä H V., Müller K, Ahokas A, Miettinen K, Rimón R, Andersson LC. Accumulation of macrophages in the CSF of schizophrenic patients during acute psychotic episodes. Am J Psychiatry. 1999;

[32] McAllister CG, Van Kammen DP, Rehn TJ, Miller AL, Gurklis J,

Kelley ME, et al. Increases in CSF levels of interleukin-2 in schizophrenia: Effects of recurrence of psychosis and medication status. Am J Psychiatry. 1995;

[33] Pathmanandavel K, Starling J, Dale RC, Brilot F. Autoantibodies and the immune hypothesis in psychotic brain diseases: Challenges and perspectives. Clinical and Developmental Immunology. 2013.

[34] Tandon R, Keshavan MS, Nasrallah HA. Schizophrenia, "Just the Facts": What we know in 2008. Part 1: Overview. Schizophr Res. 2008;

[35] Jeppesen R, Benros ME. Autoimmune diseases and psychotic disorders. Frontiers in Psychiatry. 2019.

[36] Strous RD, Shoenfeld Y. Schizophrenia, autoimmunity and immune system dysregulation: A comprehensive model updated and revisited. Journal of Autoimmunity. 2006.

[37] Lachance LR, McKenzie K. Biomarkers of gluten sensitivity in patients with non-affective psychosis: A meta-analysis. Schizophr Res. 2014;

[38] Balu DT. The NMDA Receptor and Schizophrenia. From Pathophysiology to Treatment. In: Advances in Pharmacology. 2016.

[39] Dalmau J, Lancaster E, Martinez-Hernandez E, Rosenfeld MR, Balice-Gordon R. Clinical experience and laboratory investigations in patients with anti-NMDAR encephalitis. The Lancet Neurology. 2011.

[40] Titulaer MJ, McCracken L, Gabilondo I, Armangué T, Glaser C, Iizuka T, et al. Treatment and prognostic factors for long-term outcome in patients with anti-NMDA receptor encephalitis: An observational cohort study. Lancet Neurol. 2013;

[41] Pollak TA, Lennox BR, Müller S, Benros ME, Prüss H, Tebartz van Elst L, et al. Autoimmune psychosis: an international consensus on an approach to the diagnosis and management of psychosis of suspected autoimmune origin. The Lancet Psychiatry. 2020.

[42] Ellul P, Groc L, Tamouza R, Leboyer M. The clinical challenge of autoimmune psychosis: Learning from anti-NMDA receptor autoantibodies. Frontiers in Psychiatry. 2017.

[43] Pomarol-Clotet E, Honey GD, Murray GK, Corlett PR, Absalom AR, Lee M, et al. Psychological effects of ketamine in healthy volunteers: Phenomenological study. Br J Psychiatry. 2006;

[44] Javitt DC, Zukin SR. Recent advances in the phencyclidine model of schizophrenia. Am J Psychiatry. 1991;

[45] Umbricht D, Schmid L, Koller R, Vollenweider FX, Hell D, Javitt DC. Ketamine-induced deficits in auditory and visual context-dependent processing in healthy volunteers: Implications for models of cognitive deficits in schizophrenia. Arch Gen Psychiatry. 2000;

[46] Kleckner NW, Dingledine R. Requirement for glycine in activation of NMDA receptors expressed in xenopus oocytes. Science (80-). 1988;

[47] Marsman A, Van Den Heuvel MP, Klomp DWJ, Kahn RS, Luijten PR, Hulshoff Pol HE. Glutamate in schizophrenia: A focused review and meta-analysis of 1H-MRS studies. Schizophrenia Bulletin. 2013.

[48] Bendikov I, Nadri C, Amar S, Panizzutti R, De Miranda J, Wolosker H, et al. A CSF and postmortem brain study of d-serine metabolic parameters in schizophrenia. Schizophr Res. 2007;

[49] Goltsov AY, Loseva JG, Andreeva T V., Grigorenko AP, Abramova LI,

Kaleda VG, et al. Polymorphism in the 5′-promoter region of serine racemase gene in schizophrenia. Molecular Psychiatry. 2006.

[50] Boehning D, Snyder SH. Novel neural modulators. Annual Review of Neuroscience. 2003.

[51] Bergeron R, Meyer TM, Coyle JT, Greene RW. Modulation of N-methyl-D-aspartate receptor function by glycine transport. Proc Natl Acad Sci U S A. 1998;

[52] Shams'Ili S, Grefkens J, De Leeuw B, Van den Bent M, Hooijkaas H, Van der Holt B, et al. Paraneoplastic cerebellar degeneration associated with antineuronal antibodies: Analysis of 50 patients. Brain. 2003;

[53] Dalmau J, Rosenfeld MR. Paraneoplastic syndromes of the CNS. The Lancet Neurology. 2008.

[54] Vianello M, Vitaliani R, Pezzani R, Nicolao P, Betterle C, Keir G, et al. The spectrum of antineuronal autoantibodies in a series of neurological patients. J Neurol Sci. 2004;

[55] Benyahia B, Amoura Z, Rousseau A, Le Clanche C, Carpentier A, Piette JC, et al. Paraneoplastic antineuronal antibodies in patients with systemic autoimmune diseases. J Neurooncol. 2003;

[56] Mostafa GA, Nazif HK, El-Shahawi HH, Abd El-Aziz MM, Hassan MA. Antineuronal antibodies and electroneurophysiological studies in pediatric patients with neuropsychiatric systemic lupus erythematosus. Pediatr Allergy Immunol. 2009;

[57] Mostafa GA, Al-Ayadhi LY. The relationship between the increased frequency of serum antineuronal antibodies and the severity of autism in children. Eur J Paediatr Neurol. 2012;

[58] Goines P, Haapanen L, Boyce R, Duncanson P, Braunschweig D, Delwiche L, et al. Autoantibodies to cerebellum in children with autism associate with behavior. Brain Behav Immun. 2011;

[59] Morer A, Lázaro L, Sabater L, Massana J, Castro J, Graus F. Antineuronal antibodies in a group of children with obsessive-compulsive disorder and Tourette syndrome. J Psychiatr Res. 2008;

[60] Gause C, Morris C, Vernekar S, Pardo-Villamizar C, Grados MA, Singer HS. Antineuronal antibodies in OCD: Comparisons in children with OCD-only, OCD+chronic tics and OCD+PANDAS. J Neuroimmunol. 2009;

[61] Ripke S, Neale BM, Corvin A, Walters JTR, Farh KH, Holmans PA, et al. Biological insights from 108 schizophrenia-associated genetic loci. Nature. 2014;

[62] Shi J, Levinson DF, Duan J, Sanders AR, Zheng Y, Péer I, et al. Common variants on chromosome 6p22.1 are associated with schizophrenia. Nature. 2009;

[63] Andreassen OA, Harbo HF, Wang Y, Thompson WK, Schork AJ, Mattingsdal M, et al. Genetic pleiotropy between multiple sclerosis and schizophrenia but not bipolar disorder: Differential involvement of immune-related gene loci. Mol Psychiatry. 2015;

[64] Catts VS, Lai YL, Weickert CS, Weickert TW, Catts S V. A quantitative review of the postmortem evidence for decreased cortical N-methyl-d-aspartate receptor expression levels in schizophrenia: How can we link molecular abnormalities to mismatch negativity deficits? Biol Psychol. 2016;

[65] Verrall L, Burnet PWJ, Betts JF, Harrison PJ. The neurobiology of D-amino acid oxidase and its

involvement in schizophrenia. Molecular Psychiatry. 2010.

[66] Remington G, Foussias G, Fervaha G, Agid O, Takeuchi H, Lee J, et al. Treating Negative Symptoms in Schizophrenia: an Update. Current Treatment Options in Psychiatry. 2016.

[67] Elkis H. Treatment-Resistant Schizophrenia. Psychiatric Clinics of North America. 2007.

[68] Üçok A, Gaebel W. Side effects of atypical antipsychotics: A brief overview. World Psychiatry. 2008.

[69] Laan W, Grobbee DE, Selten JP, Heijnen CJ, Kahn RS, Burger H. Adjuvant aspirin therapy reduces symptoms of schizophrenia spectrum disorders: Results from a randomized, double-blind, placebo-controlled trial. J Clin Psychiatry. 2010;

[70] Attari A, Mojdeh A, Soltani FASK, Najarzadegan MR. Aspirin inclusion in antipsychotic treatment on severity of symptoms in schizophrenia: A randimized clinical trial. Iran J Psychiatry Behav Sci. 2017;

[71] Akhondzadeh S, Tabatabaee M, Amini H, Ahmadi Abhari SA, Abbasi SH, Behnam B. Celecoxib as adjunctive therapy in schizophrenia: A double-blind, randomized and placebo-controlled trial. Schizophr Res. 2007;

[72] Rapaport MH, Delrahim KK, Bresee CJ, Maddux RE, Ahmadpour O, Dolnak D. Celecoxib augmentation of continuously Ill patients with schizophrenia. Biol Psychiatry. 2005;

[73] Berk M, Copolov D, Dean O, Lu K, Jeavons S, Schapkaitz I, et al. N-Acetyl Cysteine as a Glutathione Precursor for Schizophrenia-A Double-Blind, Randomized, Placebo-Controlled Trial. Biol Psychiatry. 2008;

[74] Farokhnia M, Azarkolah A, Adinehfar F, Khodaie-Ardakani MR, Hosseini SMR, Yekehtaz H, et al. N-acetylcysteine as an adjunct to risperidone for treatment of negative symptoms in patients with chronic schizophrenia: A randomized, double-blind, placebo-controlled study. Clin Neuropharmacol. 2013;

[75] Cryan JF, Dinan TG. Mind-altering microorganisms: The impact of the gut microbiota on brain and behaviour. Nature Reviews Neuroscience. 2012.

[76] Xiang YQ, Zheng W, Wang S Bin, Yang XH, Cai D Bin, Ng CH, et al. Adjunctive minocycline for schizophrenia: A meta-analysis of randomized controlled trials. Eur Neuropsychopharmacol. 2017;

[77] Cho M, Lee TY, Kwak Y Bin, Yoon YB, Kim M, Kwon JS. Adjunctive use of anti-inflammatory drugs for schizophrenia: A meta-analytic investigation of randomized controlled trials. Australian and New Zealand Journal of Psychiatry. 2019.

[78] Ehrenreich H, Hinze-Selch D, Stawicki S, Aust C, Knolle-Veentjer S, Wilms S, et al. Improvement of cognitive functions in chronic schizophrenic patients by recombinant human erythropoietin. Mol Psychiatry. 2007;

[79] Shen H, Li R, Yan R, Zhou X, Feng X, Zhao M, et al. Adjunctive therapy with statins in schizophrenia patients: A meta-analysis and implications. Psychiatry Res. 2018;

[80] Girgis RR, Ciarleglio A, Choo T, Haynes G, Bathon JM, Cremers S, et al. A Randomized, Double-Blind, Placebo-Controlled Clinical Trial of Tocilizumab, An Interleukin-6 Receptor Antibody, for Residual Symptoms in Schizophrenia. Neuropsychopharmacology. 2018;

[81] Miller BJ, Dias JK, Lemos HP, Buckley PF. An open-label, pilot trial of

adjunctive tocilizumab in schizophrenia. Journal of Clinical Psychiatry. 2016.

[82] Buchanan RW, Javitt DC, Marder SR, Schooler NR, Gold JM, McMahon RP, et al. The Cognitive and Negative Symptoms in Schizophrenia Trial (CONSIST): The efficacy of glutamatergic agents for negative symptoms and cognitive impairments. Am J Psychiatry. 2007;

[83] Iwata Y, Nakajima S, Suzuki T, Keefe RSE, Plitman E, Chung JK, et al. Effects of glutamate positive modulators on cognitive deficits in schizophrenia: A systematic review and meta-Analysis of double-blind randomized controlled trials. Molecular Psychiatry. 2015.

[84] Kantrowitz JT, Woods SW, Petkova E, Cornblatt B, Corcoran CM, Chen H, et al. D-serine for the treatment of negative symptoms in individuals at clinical high risk of schizophrenia: A pilot, double-blind, placebo-controlled, randomised parallel group mechanistic proof-of-concept trial. The Lancet Psychiatry. 2015;

[85] Ichim TE, Solano F, Glenn E, Morales F, Smith L, Zabrecky G, et al. Stem cell therapy for autism. J Transl Med. 2007;

[86] Weickert T, Jacomb I, Lenroot R, Lappin J, Weinberg D, Brooks W, et al. S33. REDUCTION IN PERIPHERAL C-REACTIVE PROTEIN LEVELS WITH CANAKINUMAB ADMINISTRATION IS RELATED TO REDUCED POSITIVE SYMPTOM SEVERITY IN PATIENTS WITH SCHIZOPHRENIA AND INFLAMMATION. Schizophr Bull. 2019;

[87] Raison CL, Rutherford RE, Woolwine BJ, Shuo C, Schettler P, Drake DF, et al. A randomized controlled trial of the tumor necrosis factor antagonist infliximab for treatment-resistant depression: The role of baseline inflammatory biomarkers. Arch Gen Psychiatry. 2013;

[88] Yirmiya R, Goshen I. Immune modulation of learning, memory, neural plasticity and neurogenesis. Brain Behav Immun. 2011;

[89] Harrison NA, Doeller CF, Voon V, Burgess N, Critchley HD. Peripheral inflammation acutely impairs human spatial memory via actions on medial temporal lobe glucose metabolism. Biol Psychiatry. 2014.

[90] Goldsmith DR, Rapaport MH. Inflammation and Negative Symptoms of Schizophrenia: Implications for Reward Processing and Motivational Deficits. Frontiers in Psychiatry. 2020.

[91] Vieta E, Reinares M, Rosa AR. Staging bipolar disorder. Neurotox Res. 2011;

[92] Collins SM, Surette M, Bercik P. The interplay between the intestinal microbiota and the brain. Nature Reviews Microbiology. 2012.

Chapter 6

The Role of Epigenetics in Psychosis

Esmaeil Shahsavand Ananloo

Abstract

Epigenetics (genome - environment interaction) is the study of mitotically heritable, but reversible changes in gene expression without any change in DNA modifications and the chromatin structure. Transition to psychosis is a complex and longitudinal process during which epigenetic changes have been hypothesized and investigated. This process is especially important in individuals at high/ultrahigh risk for psychosis, before the development of full-blown psychosis. Psychoses is a range of complex disorders, where genetic variants explain only a portion of risk. Neuro-epigenetic mechanisms may explain the remaining share of risk, as well as the transition from susceptibility to the actual disease. There is a need for computational model of psychosis integrating genetic risk with environmental factors (epigenetic) associated with the disorder to discover its pathophysiological pathways. Epigenetic dysregulation of many genes has been widely speculated that are important factors involved in etiology, pathophysiology, and course of the psychoses, such as schizophrenia, and mood disorders with psychotic features. In addition, the role of epigenetic changes, including histone and DNA modifications and also targeting microRNAs in the treatment of psychoses is a new field of investigations.

Keywords: psychosis, epigenetic, etiology, pathophysiology

1. Introduction

Epigenetic mechanisms, link between the environment and the genome, are known to play a major role in the structure and also physiology of the human central nervous system (CNS), such as learning, memory, circadian clock and neural plasticity [1–4]. During the last decade, a huge amount of investigations in multi-omics era, including genomics, transcriptomics, proteomics, metabolomics, lipidomics, microbiomics, epigenomics, interactomics, and connectomics have pushed brain development into the "big data" era [5–10]. Multi-directional differentiation ability and self-renewal are two primary properties that characterize embryonic stem cells [11, 12]. The major cell types in the CNS, including neurons, astrocytes, and oligodendrocytes are generated from common neural stem cells (NSC) [13, 14]. There is a large number of interdependent factors, such as epigenetic modifications, pro-inflammatory cytokines, intracellular signaling pathways, and protein complexes play important role in regulating the differentiation potential and fate specification of NSC [11, 15–17]. It is known that the epigenetic mechanisms play an important role, not only in neurogenesis during the periods of fetal life and childhood, but also in neurogenesis takes place during adulthood in the mammalian brain [18].

Recent studies highlighted that microRNAs (miRNAs) as a type of epigenetic modifications, have the pivotal role in balancing the switch from self-renewal to differentiation of embryonic stem cells (ESCs) [19]. Evidence has shown that specific circular RNA (circRNA) expression patterns are significantly associated with adult stem cell self-renewal and differentiation [17]. Epitranscriptomics (chemical modifications on RNA), including N6-methyladenosine (m^6A), 2-O-dimethyladenosine (m^6A_m), N1-methyladenosine (m^1A), 5-methylcytosine (m^5C), and isomerization of uracil to pseudouridine (Ψ) has recently garnered attention, and has biological consequences, such as embryonic stem cell differentiation, brain development, and neurodevelopmental disorders [20, 21].

In the field of mental disorders, epigenetic mechanisms are thought to play a major role in the pathogenesis of the psychoses, including schizophrenia (SCZ) and bipolar disorder (BD) [22–24].

In this review article, after a brief introduction, I will discuss around: 1) the concept of epigenetics, including its definition and applications, 2) epigenetics and psychosis, including an overview of psychosis, and short references to the roles of genetics, environment, and epigenetics in psychosis, 3) the epigenetics findings in psychosis, including a dynamic approach to psychosis, epigenetic findings in prodromal phase of psychosis, in first-episode psychosis, in overt psychosis, and in methamphetamine-induced psychosis.

2. The concept of epigenetics

2.1 Definition

In as early as 1942, Conrad Waddington (as an embryologist) first defined the field. Epigenetics means "above" or "on top of" genetics. Epigenetics is the study of mitotically heritable, but reversible, changes in gene expression that occur without a change in the genomic DNA or histone sequences, principally through modifications in chromatin structure, including DNA and histone. Epigenetics is the study of how our behaviors and environment can cause changes that affect the way our genes work.

The epigenome is a dynamic concept, and refers to the biological mechanisms, which regulate gene expression (such as DNA methylation). Although the epigenome can be altered by environmental factors, but it is stable overall [25].

2.2 Epigenetic mechanisms

These mechanisms are necessary for the regulation of gene expression and chromatin architecture at a genome-wide level in mammalian, including human cells, and play critical roles in both normal human development and disorders. Epigenetic modifications are tissue specific. There are several known mechanisms for epigenetic modification. These mechanisms are DNA and histone posttranslational modifications, including methylation, acetylation, phosphorylation, and ubiquitination, and also non-coding RNAs regulation. The methylation of DNA cytosine residues at the carbon 5 position is a common epigenetic modification that is often found in the sequence context CpG [26].

2.3 Epigenetic applications

Interest in the field of epigenetics, as well as the usage of the term, have increased significantly over the last few years [27]. Up to the January of 2021, there are 102,898 citations (29,879 reviews, 424 systematic reviews, 328 meta-analyses, and 72,267 other types of articles, including original articles) related to "epigenetics" in PubMed. In 2004, however, this number was 1017 (85 article every month), and rose to 13,125 in 2020 (1094 article every month; ~ 13 times more). In addition, there are 1,016 citations (116 reviews, 26 systematic reviews, 39 meta-analyses, and 835 other types of articles, including original articles) related to "epigenome-wide association study".

The concept of epigenetic has spread into different fields, that do not address just the genetics, such as neuroscience [28, 29], physiology [30, 31], psychiatry [32–34], addiction [35], stress [36–38], and aging [39, 40].

Complex disorders, such as endocrine, cardiovascular, skin, autoimmune, or mental disorders, result from complex interactions between genes and the environment. For example, increased DNA methylation variability may be involved in obesity [41], ischemic heart disease [42], or major depression disorder [43, 44]. Regarding the psychosis, there are 294 citations (118 reviews, 5 systematic reviews, 2 meta-analyses, and 169 other types of articles, including original articles) related to "epigenetic and psychosis", and 1058 citations (416 reviews, 13 systematic reviews, 7 meta-analyses, and 622 other types of articles, including original articles) related to "epigenetic and schizophrenia" in PubMed (accessed on January 2021).

3. Epigenetics and psychosis

3.1 An overview to psychosis

Psychotic disorders are among the frequent and disabling human disorders. In recent years, the concept of psychosis has moved from just a chronic disorder to a more dynamic paradigm. Psychosis is now conceptualized as a progressive mental disorder with transitions across several stages: early vulnerability, at-risk or ultra-high risk (UHR) mental state, first episode, and chronic disorder [25]. Schizophrenia and BD are chronic mental disorders, both considered as "major psychosis"; they are thought to share some pathogenetic factors involving dysfunctional gene x environment interactions [45]. They have heterogeneous psychiatric phenotypes, and their etiology and physiopathology still remain largely unknown [24, 46]. Psychotic disorders are highly heritable, and have polygenic inheritance underlain by pleiotropic genes [34]. So, both the genetic and environmental factors are involved in the etiology and course of the major psychoses, such as major depressive disorder (MDD), BD, and SCZ [47, 48].

3.2 An overview to the role of genetics in psychosis

Although some progress has been made in the understanding of genetic physiopathology of psychoses, and despite success in identifying cytogenetic deletions or insertions, and also genetic variants and polymorphisms associated with them, it seems that the molecular genetic findings could not yet to elucidate the exact molecular pathogenesis of different forms of psychoses [49]. Many candidate genes have been identified showing a very high genetic heterogeneity of psychoses. These genes are overrepresented in synaptic and neurotransmission pathways. Different types of common and rare genetic variants, including single nucleotide polymorphisms (SNPs) and copy number variations (CNVs) with small or large effects have also been identified in the last years. The genetic variations may impact on local DNA methylation patterns [50]. All of these findings are important in clinical practice as they can lead to therapeutic challenge or genetic counseling, but only a small fraction of psychosis could be easily explained by genetics [24].

3.3 An overview to the role of environmental factors in psychosis

Regarding the role of environmental factors in psychosis, many stressful life events, including obstetric complications, mother tobacco use during the pregnancy, and her physical inactivity, childhood trauma, emotional abuse, physical neglect, heightened sensitivity to stressful events, childhood and adolescent low functioning, affective comorbidities, male gender, single status, unemployment and low educational level have been reported [23, 51]. Trauma during the childhood mediates the epigenome and gene expression profile, and could provide a mechanism underling psychosis [22].

3.4 An overview to the role of epigenetics in psychosis

A large amount of epigenetic research in mental health was performed during the last decade. The results of these efforts have "revolutionary" potentials for the development of new interdisciplinary models of mental health [52]. Evidence show that the risk factors for psychosis were not solely due to the DNA sequence, but also abnormal epigenetic modifications have important role in the etiopathology of these disorders [53]. It has been widely speculated that a wide range of epigenetic modifications of the genome, such as DNA methylation, post-translational histone modifications (in particular the histone 3 lysine 4; H3L4), and non-coding RNAs (such as miRNAs) may mediate gene–environment interactions at the molecular level, and through transcription factors modulate the expression of psychiatric phenotypes, including the variability in symptom severity and family heritability [34, 46].

Several studies have investigated the epigenetic pattern, including DNA methylation pattern in patients with major psychosis in different tissues and associated this epigenetic modification with psychiatric phenotype [54–57]. The main hypothesis for the development of psychotic disorders, proposes that a combination of genetic and environmental factors, during critical periods of brain development, including prenatal and postnatal periods increase the risk for these disorders [46]. The epigenetic mechanisms are important heritable and dynamic means of regulating various genomic functions, including gene expression. These mechanisms orchestrate brain development, adult neurogenesis, and synaptic plasticity. These processes when perturbed are thought to contribute to psychosis, such as SCZ pathophysiology [58]. However, new epigenetic technologies may be able to uncover etiopathogenic mechanisms of major psychosis [59]. For example, There are significant differences were detected in both CpG and CpH modifications between patients with SCZ and healthy controls [59].

4. The epigenetics findings in psychosis

4.1 Epigenetics findings in prodromal phase of psychosis

The research about the complex interactions between the stressful life events with dysregulation of biological stress response systems (such as hypothalamic–pituitary–adrenal [HPA] axis) and genes; epigenetic changes; in one hand, and the initial emergence of psychosis, on the other hand, has increasingly focused on the prodromal phase of psychosis, the period of functional decline that precedes clinical illness [51]. In comparison with general population, childhood adversity rates would be higher in people at UHR of psychosis [60]. Several models, such as dysfunctional cognitive patterns, and epigenetic dysregulation have been cited to explain the link between trauma and the subsequent onset of psychosis [60].

It has been estimated that around 30 to 40% of UHR individuals convert to full-blown psychosis in the following 24 to 36 months [61]. Conversion to psychosis, especially in high and/or UHR individuals is a longitudinal process during which several epigenetic changes have been described [25]. As a few examples, it has been reported that conversion to psychosis is associated with specific methylation changes in two regions, including 1q21.1 and a cluster of six CpG regions located in glutathione s-transferase mu 5 (*GSTM5*) gene (chr1p13.3) promoter [62]. Bang et al. [63] suggest that epigenetic alterations of oxytocin receptor (*OXTR*) gene, located on chromosome 3 (chr3p25.3) can be detected before the development of full-blown psychosis (**Table 1**).

Chromosomal region	Gene	Epigenetic modification	Reference
chr1p13.3	glutathione s-transferase mu 5 (*GSTM5*); six CpG regions	Methylation	[62]
Two regions of chr1q21.1	Intergenic	Methylation	[62]
chr3p25.3	oxytocin receptor (*OXTR*)	Methylation	[63]

Table 1.
An overview to the epigenetic studies in prodromal phase of psychosis.

4.2 Epigenetics findings in first-episode psychosis

The onset of psychosis is the result of complex interactions between genetic vulnerability to psychosis and response to environmental and/or developmental changes. Epigenetic modifications mediate the interplay between genes and environment leading to the onset of psychosis [62]. It has been hypothesized that the neural diathesis-stress model proposes that different stressors act on a pre-existing vulnerability and thus triggers the presenting symptoms of psychosis [64].

The global DNA hypomethylation; increased methylation and reduced gene expression of GTP cyclohydrolase 1 (*GCH1*, located on chromosome 14 [chr14q22.2]), hyperexpression of udE neurodevelopmental protein 1 like 1 (*NDEL1*, located on chromosome 17 [chr17p13.1]), AKT serine/threonine kinase 1 (*AKT1*, located on chromosome 14 [chr14q32.33]), DICER1 antisense RNA1 (*DICER1*, located on chromosome 14 [chr14q32.13]), and hypoexpression of drosha ribonuclease III (*DROSHA*, located on chromosome 5 [chr5p13.3]), catechol-O-methyltransferase (*COMT*, located on chromosome 22 [chr22q11.21]), and disturbed in schizophrenia 1 (*DISC1*, located on chromosome 1 [chr1q42.2]) have all been reported in first-episode psychosis [22].

Hypomethylation has been founded among all CpGs analyzed within the promoter of glutamate ionotropic receptor NMDA type subunit 2B (*GRIN2B*) gene, located on chromosome 12 (chr12p13.1) in patients with first-episode patients with SCZ and greater LINE-1 type transposase domain-containing protein 1 (*L1TD1P1*) gene, located on chromosome 1 (chr1p31.3) methylation in patients and their siblings [65].

Human endogenous retroviruses (HERV) have been widely associated with the etiology of SCZ. The lower endogenous retroviral sequence K 2 (*ERVK2*, located on chromosome 19 [chr19q11]) methylation levels have been reported at early stages of SCZ [66].

Chromosomal region	Gene	Epigenetic modification	Reference
chr14q22.2	GTP cyclohydrolase 1 (GCH1)	Hypermethylation	[22]
chr17p13.1	udE neurodevelopmental protein 1 like 1 (*NDEL1*)	Hyperexpression	[22]
chr14q32.33	AKT serine/threonine kinase 1 (*AKT1*)	Hyperexpression	[22]
chr14q32.13	DICER1 antisense RNA1 (*DICER1*)	Hyperexpression	[22]
chr5p13.3	drosha ribonuclease III (*DROSHA*)	Hypoexpression	[22]
chr22q11.21	catechol-O-methyltransferase (*COMT*)	Hypoexpression	[22]
chr13q33.1	disturbed in schizophrenia 1 (*DISC1*)	Hypoexpression	[22]
chr12p13.1	glutamate ionotropic receptor NMDA type subunit 2B (*GRIN2B*)	Hypomethylation	[65]
chr1q42.2	LINE-1 type transposase domain-containing protein 1 (*L1TD1P1*)	Hyperexpression	[65]
chr19q11	endogenous retroviral sequence K 2 (*ERVK2*)	Hypomethylation	[66]
chr12p13.1	glutamate ionotropic receptor NMDA type subunit 2B (*GRIN2B*)	Hyperexpression	[67]

Table 2.
An overview to the epigenetic studies in first episode psychosis.

Working memory and executive functions impairments emerge in first-episode psychosis, and even prior to its onset. It has been reported that NMDA receptor hypofunction is a feature of early postnatal development, with epigenetic hyper-repression of the glutamate ionotropic receptor NMDA type subunit 2B (*GRIN2B*), located on chromosome 12 (chr12p13.1) promoter being a contributing factor. This loss of NR2B protein may induce synaptic dysfunctions during development and may underlie early cognitive impairments in patients with SCZ (**Table 2**) [67].

4.3 Epigenetics findings in overt psychosis

Although numerous studies have examined psychosis-associated gene expression changes, epigenetic studies of psychosis are in their infancy [55]. For example, it seems that DNA methylation plays an important role in SCZ; directly as a mechanism of pathogenesis or as a risk biomarker [68]. Different epigenetic modifications have been reported in psychosis, genes implicated in dopaminergic, serotonergic, GABAergic and glutamatergic pathways [45, 46]. Specific changes in promoter DNA methylation activity of genes related to SCZ such as reelin, BDNF and GAD67, and altered expression and function of mGlu2/3 receptors in the frontal cortex have been reported [45].

Abnormal neuronal processes, including dopamine imbalance, may be the central to the pathogenesis of major psychosis. DNA methylation, transcriptomic, and genetic-epigenetic interactions in major psychosis converged on pathways of neurodevelopment, synaptic activity, and immune functions [69]. It has been suggested that hypomethylation of the enhancer at insulin-like growth factor 2 (*IGF2*, located on chromosome 11 [chr11p15.5]) may enhance dopamine synthesis associated with major psychosis. This enhancer targets the nearby tyrosine hydroxylase (*TH*, located on chromosome 11 [chr11p15.5]) responsible for dopamine synthesis [69].

Walton et al. [70] suggest that epigenetic alterations (DNA methylation) in genes implicated in neurodevelopment (such as Sp6 transcription factor; [*SP6*] gene, located on chromosome 17 [chr17q21.32]) may contribute to a brain-based biomarker (amygdala/hippocampal volume ratio) of psychotic psychopathology.

Reelin (RELN) is a large secreted extracellular matrix glycoprotein that helps regulate processes of neuronal migration and positioning in the developing brain by controlling cell–cell interactions [71]. Reelin located on chromosome 7 (chr7q22.1) is one of the most frequently studied candidates in methylation studies of SCZ [26]. Reelin is mostly synthesized in GABAergic neurons of corticolimbic structures. Reelin binds to AUP1 lipid droplet regulating VLDL assembly factor (*AUP1*, located on chromosome 2 [chr2p13.1]), apolipoprotein E (*APOE*, located on chromosome 19 [chr19q13.32]), and α3β2 Integrin receptors located on dendritic shafts and spines of postsynaptic pyramidal neurons. It has been shown that altered *RELN* expression in patients with SCZ and BD patients is associated with altered epigenetic homeostasis [72].

The loss of the human brain regions laterality (such as in temporal lobe, basal ganglia and white matter microstructure) is one of the most consistent modalities in SCZ and BD [73–75]. This loss of brain laterality corresponds to aberrant epigenetic regulation of transforming growth factor beta 2 (*TGFB2*, located on chromosome 1 [chr1q41]) and changes in transforming growth factor beta superfamily (TGFβ) signaling [76]. These findings may be potential avenues for disorders prevention/treatment.

In their metagenome-wide association study (MWAS), Aberg et al. [26] found that MINDY2 lysine 48 deubiquitinase 2 (*MINDY2*, located on chromosome 15 [chr15q21.3-q22.1]), a part of the networks regulated by microRNA (as an epigenetic regulator), is linked to neuronal differentiation and dopaminergic gene expression [77–79], that has potential relevance to SCZ.

Epigenetic alterations of oxytocin receptor (*OXTR*) gene, (located on chromosome 3 [chr3p25.3]) occur across psychotic disorders. It has been reported that patients with SCZ (especially in women) show higher levels of DNA methylation. This pattern of *OXTR* methylation is associated with poorer emotion recognition, smaller volumes in temporal-limbic and prefrontal regions [80].

Discoidin domain receptor 1 (*DDR1*) gene is located on chromosome 6 (chr6p21.33). *DDR1* hypermethylation has been found in patients with psychosis. This hypermethylation is associated with mental stress, and neutrophil-to-lymphocyte ratios [81].

The brain parvalbumin deficits are a consistent finding in SCZ and models of psychosis. Greater methylation of parvalbumin (*PVALB*) gene, located on chromosome 22 (chr22q12.3) is found in hippocampus of the patients with SCZ. The LINE-1 type transposase domain-containing protein 1 (*L1TD1P1*) gene methylation, as a measure of global methylation, is also elevated in both regions of hippocampus and prefrontal cortex in SCZ [82].

Associations between altered DNA methylation of the serotonin transporter-encoding gene (*SLC6A4*, located on chromosome 17 [chr17q11.2]), and early life events, and mood disorders have been reported. Childhood trauma exposure may be a robust environmental risk factor for psychosis. However, not all exposed individuals develop psychotic symptoms later in life [83]. Hypermethylation of the CpG site in *SLC6A4* is involved in the pathophysiology of SCZ, especially in male patients harboring low-activity 5-HTTLPR alleles [84].

Histone deacetylases (HDACs) are enzymes that regulate cognitive circuitry. HDAC expression positively correlate with cognitive performance scores [85]. Postmortem brain studies support dysregulated expression of the histone deacetylase enzymes, HDAC1 and HDAC2, as a central feature in disorders, including SCZ

Chromosomal region	Gene	Epigenetic modification	Reference
chr11p15.5	insulin-like growth factor 2 (*IGF2*)	Hypermethylation	[69]
chr17q21.32	Sp6 transcription factor; (*SP6*)	Hypermethylation	[70]
chr7q22.1	Reelin (*RELN*)	Hypoexpression	[72]
chr1q41	transforming growth factor beta 2 (*TGFB2*)	Hypoexpression	[76]
chr15q21.3-q22.1	MINDY2 lysine 48 deubiquitinase 2 (*MINDY2*)	Hypoexpression	[77–79]
chr3p25.3	oxytocin receptor (*OXTR*) gene	Hypermethylation	[80]
chr6p21.33	discoidin domain receptor 1 (*DDR1*)	Hypermethylation	[81]
chr22q12.3	parvalbumin (*PVALB*)	Hypermethylation	[82]
chr1q42.2	LINE-1 type transposase domain-containing protein 1 (*L1TD1P1*)	Hypermethylation	[65]
chr17q11.2	serotonin transporter-encoding gene (*SLC6A4*)	Hypermethylation	[83, 84]
chr1p35.2-p35.1	histone deacetylase 1 (*HDAC1*)	Hypoexpression	[85]
Chr6q21	histone deacetylase 2 (*HDAC2*)	Hypoexpression	[85]

Table 3.
An overview to the epigenetic studies in overt psychosis.

and BD [86]. It has been reported that HDAC expression is lower in the dorsolateral prefrontal cortex (DLPFC) and orbitofrontal gyrus, and higher relative HDAC expression in the cerebral white matter, pons, and cerebellum of patients with SCZ (**Table 3**) [85].

In utero exposure to diethylstilbestrol (DES), psychosis is associated with specific methylomic modifications that could impact neurodevelopment and neuroplasticity [87].

It seems that the neuronal synapses are fundamental units of mental activities. Despite the diverse origins of specific molecular dysfunctions of mental disorders, disruption of synaptic regulation, which is fundamental to behavioral adaptation to the environment, is so important. A novel class of molecular regulators of fine synaptic tuning known as long non-coding RNA (lncRNA) operates as epigenetic modifiers and enhancers of proteome diversity [88]. Non-coding RNAs, including specific microRNAs and lncRNAs provide a novel and complex mechanism of gene regulation [89]. Evidence shows remarkable alterations of the expression of lncRNAs in mental disorders, such as SCZ, suggesting the disruption of fine synaptic tuning underlying psychosis [88].

4.4 Epigenetics findings in methamphetamine-induced psychosis

Methamphetamine (MAP) causes severe substance dependence and psychosis, similar to SCZ, through the alterations in gene expression [90]. Evidence shows that epigenetic factors may play important role in methamphetamine psychosis. Nohesara et al. [91] found statistically significant DNA hypomethylation of the promoter regions of dopamine receptor D3 (*DRD3*, located on chromosome 3 [chr3q13.31]), dopamine receptor D4 (*DRD4*, located on chromosome 11 [chr11p15.5]), *MB-COMT*, and *AKT1* associated with increased expression of the corresponding genes in patients with methamphetamine psychosis. It is suggested

Chromosomal region	Gene	Epigenetic modification	Reference
chr3q13.31	dopamine receptor D3 (*DRD3*)	Hypomethylation	[90]
chr11p15.5	dopamine receptor D4 (*DRD4*)	Hypomethylation	[90]
chr22q11.21	catechol-O-methyltransferase (*COMT*)	Hyperexpression	[90]
chr14q32.33	AKT serine/threonine kinase 1 (*AKT1*)	Hyperexpression	[90]
chr7q22.1	Reelin (*RELN*)	Hypoexpression	[89]
chr10p13	tRNA aspartic acid methyltransferase 1 (*TRDMT1*)	Hypoexpression	[89]

Table 4.
An overview to the epigenetic studies in methamphetamine-induced psychosis.

that MAP can alter DNA methylation of *RELN* and tRNA aspartic acid methyltransferase 1 (*TRDMT1*, located on chromosome 10 [chr10p13]) genes in hippocampus dentate gyrus, and decrease in *RELN* mRNA in the frontal cortex. These alterations might be related to SCZ-like psychotic symptoms of MAP psychosis (**Table 4**) [90].

5. Summary and future directions

5.1 Summary

In this review article, after a brief introduction, I discussed the concepts of psychosis and epigenetics, and also references to the roles of genetics, environment, and epigenetics in psychosis. In addition, I mentioned the epigenetics findings in prodromal phase of psychosis, first-episode psychosis, overt psychosis, and also in methamphetamine-induced psychosis.

Psychotic disorders, such as SCZ and BD are among the frequent, disabling, progressive, and chronic human mental disorders, and have heterogeneous psychiatric phenotypes. Psychosis has several stages, including early vulnerability, at-risk or ultra-high risk mental state, first episode, and chronic disorder. It seems that dysfunctional genes x environment interactions influence their pathogenesis. Psychotic disorders are highly heritable, and have a polygenic inheritance pattern. Despite success in identifying cytogenetic changes, many candidate genes in synaptic and neurotransmission pathways, and also genetic polymorphisms, including SNPs and CNVs associated with psychosis, the molecular genetic findings could not yet explain its exact molecular pathogenesis. Although all of these findings are important in clinical practice, such as therapeutic challenge or genetic counseling, but only a small fraction of psychosis could be easily explained by genetics. However, the genetic variants explain only a portion of risk, and the epigenetic mechanisms may explain the remaining share of risk. In addition, many stressful environmental factors, such as obstetric complications, childhood trauma, different forms of child abuse or neglect have also been reported to play roles in the association with psychosis. These factors mediate the epigenetic modifications, and could provide a mechanism underling psychosis.

Epigenetics means "above" or "on top of" genetics. It refers to the biological mechanisms, which regulate gene expression. Epigenetics is the study of reversible changes in gene expression without any change in chromatin structure. The DNA methylation of cytosine residues at the carbon 5 position is a common epigenetic modification. Interest in the field of epigenetics has increased significantly over the last few years. It plays a key role in the structure and also physiology of the human CNS, and also in the development of complex disorders, such as endocrine, cardiovascular, skin, autoimmune, and mental disorders. Epigenetic mechanisms, including DNA and histone modifications, and also non-coding RNAs are especially important mechanisms to detect the people with high/ultrahigh risk for psychosis.

A large amount of epigenetic research in mental health was performed during the last years, and these efforts have "revolutionary" potentials for the development of new interdisciplinary models of mental health. The main hypothesis for the development of psychotic disorders, proposes that a combination of genetic, environmental, and developmental factors increase the risk for these disorders. It has been widely speculated that a wide range of epigenetic modifications of the genome may mediate gene–environment interactions and modulate the expression of psychiatric phenotypes. There are some epigenetic dysregulations in prodromal phase of psychosis, to find the people at UHR of psychosis. During the conversion to psychosis, especially in high and/or UHR individuals, several epigenetic changes have also been described. Epigenetics findings in first-episode psychosis shows that the epigenetic modifications of many genes lead to the onset of psychosis. In addition, numerous studies have examined many psychosis-associated gene expression changes in overt psychosis, including methamphetamine-induced psychosis. For example, several epigenetic modifications in genes implicated in dopaminergic, serotonergic, GABAergic and glutamatergic pathways, have been reported in psychosis.

5.2 Future directions

Attempting to predict future is so difficult. This is particularly true in the field of psychiatry. This in mainly due to essential deficiencies in understanding the etiopathogenesis of mental disorders. For example, mapping the relationship between human epigenetics and mental and psychiatric phenotypes is a challenging task. It is essential to shift paradigm in understanding the etiology and pathophysiology of different forms of psychosis.

During the last years, a large amount of studies in multi-omics era have pushed brain development into the "big data" era, and may promise to answer major questions of psychiatry [92]. Nowadays, there are available web-based tools for integration and interpretation of omics data. Although a large amount of studies has been performed and significant progress has been made in past years, different factors, including the high heritability, clinical heterogeneity (etiological and symptomatological), and genetic and epigenetic heterogeneity of psychosis still post as major challenges to the epigenetic dissection of this complex syndrome. However, understanding of epigenetic mechanisms is important to understand the pathogenic pathways in complex disorders, including psychosis [93]. The epigenetic studies could represent a promising approach to better understanding and treating mental disorders. The methylation modifications may be used as diagnostic markers of disorder phenotype and predict the progression and response to treatment. So, the targeted epigenetic pharmacotherapy, in combination with other types of effective interventions, will be effective for future personalized psychiatry for patients [94].

Despite significant progress in identifying the mechanisms underlying psychosis, there are no valid biomarkers for both disorder phenotyping and treatment response. It seems that psychiatric diagnosis based on biomarkers will be more valid and reliable than symptoms-based diagnosis. The discovery of biomarkers, such as epigenetic biomarkers in mental disorders will help in the prevention, diagnosis, and treatment of patients with these disorders [95]. DNA methylation may play an important role in psychosis as a biomarker of risk. Blood DNA-methylation signatures show promise of serving as a biomarker of SCZ [96]. However, the sensitivity and stability of epigenetic alterations in specific genes make them promising candidates for robust biomarkers [94, 97].

Finally, there is a need for computational model of psychosis integrating genetic risk with environmental, and developmental factors associated with the disorder to discover its pathophysiological pathways, and more accurate treatment targets for psychosis. Hopefully, the epigenetics may provide new insights into a more comprehensive interpretation of mental disorders, such as psychosis and might eventually improve the nosology, treatment, and prevention of these complex disorders.

Author details

Esmaeil Shahsavand Ananloo
Department of Psychosomatic, Imam Khomeini Hospital Complex (IKHC), School of Medicine, Tehran University of Medical Sciences (TUMS), Tehran, Iran

*Address all correspondence to: shahsavand@tums.ac.ir; esmaeilshahsavand@gmail.com

References

[1] Jiang Y, Langley B, Lubin FD, Renthal W, Wood MA, Yasui DH, Kumar A, Nestler EJ, Akbarian S, Beckel-Mitchener AC. Epigenetics in the nervous system. Journal of Neuroscience. 2008 28 (46):11753-11759. DOI: 10.1523/JNEUROSCI.3797-08.2008

[2] Borrelli E, Nestler EJ, Allis CD, Sassne-Corsi P. Decoding the epigenetic language of neuronal plasticity. Neuron. 2008 Dec 26;60(6):961-974. DOI: 10.1016/j.neuron.2008.10.012

[3] Masri S, Sassone-Corsi P. Plasticity and specificity of the circadian epigenome. Nature neuroscience. 2010 13 (11):1324. DOI: 10.1038/nn.2668

[4] Peedicayil J. Epigenetic management of major psychosis. Clinical epigenetics. 2011 Aug 1;2(2):249-256. DOI: 10.1007/s13148-011-0038-2

[5] Geerts H, Dacks PA, Devanarayan V, Haas M, Khachaturian ZS, Gordon MF, Maudsley S, Romero K, Stephenson D, Brain Health Modeling Initiative. Big data to smart data in Alzheimer's disease: The brain health modeling initiative to foster actionable knowledge. Alzheimer's & Dementia. 2016 Sep 1;12(9):1014-1021. DOI: 10.1016/j.jalz.2016.04.008

[6] Alonso-Betanzos A, Bolón-Canedo V. Big-data analysis, cluster analysis, and machine-learning approaches. InSex-Specific Analysis of Cardiovascular Function 2018 (pp. 607-626). Springer, Cham. DOI: 10.1007/978-3-319-77932-4_37

[7] Mayer EA, Labus J, Aziz Q, Tracey I, Kilpatrick L, Elsenbruch S, Schweinhardt P, Van Oudenhove L, Borsook D. Role of brain imaging in disorders of brain–gut interaction: a Rome Working Team Report. Gut. 2019 Sep 1;68(9):1701-1715. DOI: 10.1136/gutjnl-2019-318308

[8] Pralle RS, White HM. Symposium review: Big data, big predictions: Utilizing milk Fourier-transform infrared and genomics to improve hyperketonemia management. Journal of Dairy Science. 2020 Apr 1;103(4):3867-3873. DOI: 10.3168/jds.2019-17379

[9] Briscoe J, Marín O. Looking at neurodevelopment through a big data lens. Science. 2020 Sep 18;369(6510). DOI: 10.1126/science.aaz8627

[10] Jourdon A, Scuderi S, Capauto D, Abyzov A, Vaccarino FM. PsychENCODE and beyond: transcriptomics and epigenomics of brain development and organoids. Neuropsychopharmacology. 2021 Jan;46(1):70-85. DOI: 10.1038/s41386-020-0763-3

[11] Mohamed Ariff I, Mitra A, Basu A. Epigenetic regulation of self-renewal and fate determination in neural stem cells. Journal of neuroscience research. 2012 Mar;90(3):529-539. DOI: 10.1002/jnr.22804

[12] Chen G, Guo YE, Li C, Li S, Wan X. Small Molecules that Promote Self-Renewal of Stem Cells and Somatic Cell Reprogramming. Stem Cell Reviews and Reports. 2020 Mar 17:1-3. DOI: 10.1007/s12015-020-09965-w

[13] Namihira M, Kohyama J, Abematsu M, Nakashima K. Epigenetic mechanisms regulating fate specification of neural stem cells. Philosophical Transactions of the Royal Society B: Biological Sciences. 2008 Jun 27;363(1500):2099-2109. DOI: 10.1098/rstb.2008.2262

[14] Sanosaka T, Namihira M, Nakashima K. Epigenetic mechanism in sequential differentiation of neural stem cells. Epigenetics. 2009 Feb 16;4(2):89-92. DOI: 10.4161/epi.4.2.8233

[15] Jahandideh B, Derakhshani M, Abbaszadeh H, Movassaghpour AA, Mehdizadeh A, Talebi M, Yousefi M. The pro-Inflammatory cytokines effects on mobilization, self-renewal and differentiation of hematopoietic stem cells. Human Immunology. 2020 Mar 2. DOI: 10.1016/j.humimm.2020.01.004

[16] Semba T, Sammons R, Wang X, Xie X, Dalby KN, Ueno NT. JNK Signaling in Stem Cell Self-Renewal and Differentiation. International Journal of Molecular Sciences. 2020 Jan;21(7):2613. DOI: 10.3390/ijms21072613

[17] Wang Y, Jiang Z, Yu M, Yang G. Roles of circular RNAs in regulating the self-renewal and differentiation of adult stem cells. Differentiation. 2020 Mar 6. DOI: 10.1016/j.diff.2020.03.001

[18] Ma DK, Marchetto MC, Guo JU, Ming GL, Gage FH, Song H. Epigenetic choreographers of neurogenesis in the adult mammalian brain. Nature neuroscience. 2010 13 (11):1338-1344. DOI: 10.1038/nn.2672

[19] Divisato G, Passaro F, Russo T, Parisi S. The Key Role of MicroRNAs in Self-Renewal and Differentiation of Embryonic Stem Cells. International Journal of Molecular Sciences. 2020 Jan;21(17):6285. DOI: 10.3390/ijms21176285

[20] Yoon KJ, Ringeling FR, Vissers C, Jacob F, Pokrass M, Jimenez-Cyrus D, Su Y, Kim NS, Zhu Y, Zheng L, Kim S. Temporal control of mammalian cortical neurogenesis by m6A methylation. Cell. 2017 Nov 2;171(4):877-889. DOI: 10.1016/j.nbd.2020.105139

[21] Vissers C, Sinha A, Ming GL, Song H. The epitranscriptome in stem cell biology and neural development. Neurobiology of Disease. 2020 Oct 13:105139. DOI: 10.1016/j.nbd.2020.105139

[22] Tomassi S, Tosato S. Epigenetics and gene expression profile in first-episode psychosis: The role of childhood trauma. Neuroscience & Biobehavioral Reviews. 2017 Dec 1;83:226-237. DOI: 10.1016/j.neubiorev.2017.10.018

[23] Fusar-Poli P, Tantardini M, De Simone S, Ramella-Cravaro V, Oliver D, Kingdon J, Kotlicka-Antczak M, Valmaggia L, Lee J, Millan MJ, Galderisi S. Deconstructing vulnerability for psychosis: Meta-analysis of environmental risk factors for psychosis in subjects at ultra high-risk. European Psychiatry. 2017 Feb;40:65-75. DOI: 10.1016/j.eurpsy.2016.09.003

[24] Chaumette B, Kebir Q, Krebs MO. Genetics and epigenetics of schizophrenia and other psychoses. Biol Aujourdhui. 2017 211 (1):69-82. DOI: 10.1051/jbio/2017015

[25] Kebir O, Chaumette B, Krebs MO. Epigenetic variability in conversion to psychosis: novel findings from an innovative longitudinal methylomic analysis. Translational psychiatry. 2018 Apr 26;8(1):1-0. DOI: 10.1038/s41398-018-0138-2

[26] Aberg KA, McClay JL, Nerella S, Clark S, Kumar G, Chen W, Khachane AN, Xie L, Hudson A, Gao G, Harada A. Methylome-wide association study of schizophrenia: identifying blood biomarker signatures of environmental insults. JAMA psychiatry. 2014 Mar 1;71(3):255-264. DOI: 10.1001/jamapsychiatry.2013.3730

[27] Deans C, Maggert KA. What do you mean,"epigenetic"?. Genetics. 2015 Apr 1;199(4):887-896. DOI: 10.1534/genetics.114.173492

[28] Calvey T, Howells FM. An introduction to psychedelic neuroscience. InProgress in Brain

Research 2018 Jan 1 (Vol. 242, pp. 1-23). Elsevier. DOI: 10.1016/bs.pbr.2018.09.013

[29] Salinas RD, Connolly DR, Song H. Invited Review: Epigenetics in neurodevelopment. Neuropathology and Applied Neurobiology. 2020 Feb;46(1):6-27. DOI: 10.1111/nan.12608

[30] Panni S, Lovering RC, Porras P, Orchard S. Non-coding RNA regulatory networks. Biochimica et Biophysica Acta (BBA)-Gene Regulatory Mechanisms. 2020 Jun 1;1863(6):194417. DOI: 10.1016/j.bbagrm.2019.194417

[31] Ho DH, Burggren WW. Epigenetics and transgenerational transfer: a physiological perspective. Journal of Experimental Biology. 2010 Jan 1;213(1):3-16. DOI: 10.1242/jeb.019752

[32] Dąbek A, Wojtala M, Pirola L, Balcerczyk A. Modulation of Cellular Biochemistry, Epigenetics and Metabolomics by Ketone Bodies. Implications of the Ketogenic Diet in the Physiology of the Organism and Pathological States. Nutrients. 2020 Mar;12(3):788. DOI: 10.3390/nu12030788

[33] Dai Z, Ramesh V, Locasale JW. The evolving metabolic landscape of chromatin biology and epigenetics. Nature Reviews Genetics. 2020 Dec;21(12):737-753. DOI: 10.1038/s41576-020-0270-8

[34] Smigielski L, Jagannath V, Rössler W, Walitza S, Grünblatt E. Epigenetic mechanisms in schizophrenia and other psychotic disorders: a systematic review of empirical human findings. Molecular Psychiatry. 2020 Jan 6:1-31. DOI: 10.1038/s41380-019-0601-3

[35] Hamilton PJ, Nestler EJ. Epigenetics and addiction. Current opinion in neurobiology. 2019 Dec 1;59:128-136. DOI: 10.1016/j.conb.2019.05.005

[36] Lemche E. Early life stress and epigenetics in late-onset Alzheimer's dementia: a systematic review. Current genomics. 2018 Nov 1;19(7):522-602. DOI: 10.2174/1389202919666171229145156

[37] Zannas AS. Epigenetics as a key link between psychosocial stress and aging: concepts, evidence, mechanisms. Dialogues in Clinical Neuroscience. 2019 Dec;21(4):389. DOI: 10.31887/DCNS.2019.21.4/azannas

[38] Cao-Lei L, De Rooij SR, King S, Matthews SG, Metz GA, Roseboom TJ, Szyf M. Prenatal stress and epigenetics. Neuroscience & Biobehavioral Reviews. 2017 May 18. DOI: 10.1016/j.neubiorev.2017.05.016

[39] Unnikrishnan A, Freeman WM, Jackson J, Wren JD, Porter H, Richardson A. The role of DNA methylation in epigenetics of aging. Pharmacology & therapeutics. 2019 Mar 1;195:172-185. DOI: 10.1016/j.pharmthera.2018.11.001

[40] Zhang W, Qu J, Liu GH, Belmonte JC. The ageing epigenome and its rejuvenation. Nature reviews Molecular cell biology. 2020 Feb 4:1-4. DOI: 10.1038/s41580-019-0204-5

[41] Xu X, Su S, Barnes VA, De Miguel C, Pollock J, Ownby D, Shi H, Zhu H, Snieder H, Wang X. A genome-wide methylation study on obesity: differential variability and differential methylation. Epigenetics. 2013 May 1;8(5):522-533. DOI: 10.4161/epi.24506

[42] Agha G, Mendelson MM, Ward-Caviness CK, Joehanes R, Huan T, Gondalia R, Salfati E, Brody JA, Fiorito G, Bressler J, Chen BH. Blood leukocyte DNA methylation predicts risk of future myocardial infarction and coronary heart disease: a longitudinal

study of 11 461 participants from population-based cohorts. Circulation. 2019 Aug 20;140(8):645-657. DOI: 10.1161/CIRCULATIONAHA.118.039357

[43] Byrne EM, Carrillo-Roa T, Henders AK, Bowdler L, McRae AF, Heath AC, Martin NG, Montgomery GW, Krause L, Wray NR. Monozygotic twins affected with major depressive disorder have greater variance in methylation than their unaffected co-twin. Translational psychiatry. 2013 Jun;3(6):e269. DOI: 10.1038/tp.2013.45

[44] Oh G, Wang SC, Pal M, Chen ZF, Khare T, Tochigi M, Ng C, Yang YA, Kwan A, Kaminsky ZA, Mill J. DNA modification study of major depressive disorder: beyond locus-by-locus comparisons. Biological psychiatry. 2015 Feb 1;77(3):246-255. DOI: 10.1016/j.biopsych.2014.06.016

[45] Matrisciano F, Panaccione I, R Grayson D, Nicoletti F, Guidotti A. Metabotropic glutamate 2/3 receptors and epigenetic modifications in psychotic disorders: a review. Current neuropharmacology. 2016 Jan 1;14(1):41-47. DOI: 10.2174/1570159x13666150713174242

[46] Rivollier F, Lotersztajn L, Chaumette B, Kebir KO. Epigenetics of schizophrenia: a review. Encephale. 2014 Oct;40(5):380-386. DOI: 10.1016/j.encep.2014.06.005

[47] Goto Y, Lee YA, Yamaguchi Y, Jas E. Biological mechanisms underlying evolutionary origins of psychotic and mood disorders. Neuroscience research 2016 (111):13-24. DOI: 10.1016/j.neures.2016.04.007

[48] Kircher T, Wöhr M, Nenadic I, Schwarting R, Schratt G, Alferink J, Culmsee C, Garn H, Hahn T, Müller-Myhsok B, Dempfle A. Neurobiology of the major psychoses: a translational perspective on brain structure and function—the FOR2107 consortium. European archives of psychiatry and clinical neuroscience. 2019 Dec 1;269(8):949-962. DOI: 10.1007/s00406-018-0943-x

[49] Hannon E, Dempster E, Burrage J, McQuillin A, Clair DS, Morris D, Di Forti M, Gaughran F, MacCabe J, Breen G, Collier D. AN INTEGRATED GENETIC-EPIGENETIC ANALYSIS OF SCHIZOPHRENIA: EVIDENCE FOR CO-LOCALIZATION OF GENETIC ASSOCIATIONS AND DIFFERENTIAL DNA METHYLATION FROM A LARGE META-ANALYSIS OF WHOLE BLOOD DNA. European Neuropsycho pharmacology. 2019 Jan 1;29:S782-3. DOI: 10.1186/s13059-016-1041-x

[50] Alfimova M, Kondratyev N, Golov A, Golimbet V. Relationship between Alzheimer's disease-associated SNPs within the CLU gene, local DNA methylation and episodic verbal memory in healthy and schizophrenia subjects. Psychiatry Research. 2019 Feb 1;272:380-386. DOI: 10.1016/j.psychres.2018.12.134

[51] W Holtzman C, I Shapiro D, D Trotman H, F Walker E. Stress and the prodromal phase of psychosis. Current pharmaceutical design. 2012 Feb 1;18(4):527-533. DOI: 10.2174/138161212799316280

[52] Cromby J, Chung E, Papadopoulos D, Talbot C. Reviewing the epigenetics of schizophrenia. Journal of Mental Health. 2019 Jan 2;28(1):71-79. DOI: 10.1080/09638237.2016.1207229

[53] Gürel Ç, Kuşçu GC, Yavaşoğlu A, Avcı ÇB. The Clues in Solving The Mystery of Major Psychosis: The Epigenetic Basis of Schizophrenia and Bipolar Disorder. Neuroscience & Biobehavioral Reviews. 2020 Mar 5. DOI: 10.1016/j.neubiorev.2020.03.005

[54] Dempster EL, Pidsley R, Schalkwyk LC, Owens S, Georgiades A,

Kane F, Kalidindi S, et al. Disease-associated epigenetic changes in monozygotic twins discordant for schizophrenia and bipolar disorder. Human molecular genetics 2011 20 (24):4786-4796. DOI: 10.1093/hmg/ddr416

[55] Pidsley R, Mill J. Epigenetic studies of psychosis: current findings, methodological approaches, and implications for postmortem research. Biological psychiatry. 2011 Jan 15;69(2):146-156. DOI: 10.1016/j.biopsych.2010.03.029

[56] Chen C, Zhang C, Cheng L, Reilly JL, Bishop JR, Sweeney JA, Chen HY, Gershon ES, Liu C. Correlation between DNA methylation and gene expression in the brains of patients with bipolar disorder and schizophrenia. Bipolar disorders 2014 16, (8):790-799. DOI: 10.1111/bdi.12255

[57] Ruzicka WB, Subburaju S, Benes FM. Circuit-and diagnosis-specific DNA methylation changes at γ-aminobutyric acid–related genes in postmortem human hippocampus in schizophrenia and bipolar disorder. JAMA psychiatry. 2015 Jun 1;72(6):541-551. DOI: 10.1001/jamapsychiatry.2015.49

[58] Whitton L, Cosgrove D, Clarkson C, Harold D, Kendall K, Richards A, Mantripragada K, Owen MJ, O'Donovan MC, Walters J, Hartmann A. Cognitive analysis of schizophrenia risk genes that function as epigenetic regulators of gene expression. American Journal of Medical Genetics Part B: Neuropsychiatric Genetics. 2016 Dec;171(8):1170-1179. DOI: 10.1002/ajmg.b.32503

[59] Pal M, Ebrahimi S, Oh G, Khare T, Zhang A, Kaminsky ZA, Wang SC, Petronis A. High precision DNA modification analysis of HCG9 in major psychosis. Schizophrenia bulletin. 2016 Jan 1;42(1):170-177. DOI: 10.1093/schbul/sbv079

[60] Fekih-Romdhane F, Ben FS, Hakiri A, Cheour M. Childhood trauma in subjects at ultra high risk for psychosis. Presse medicale (Paris, France: 1983). 2019 Mar;48(3 Pt 1):243. DOI: 10.1016/j.lpm.2018.11.023

[61] Fusar-Poli P, Borgwardt S, Bechdolf A, Addington J, Riecher-Rössler A, Schultze-Lutter F, Keshavan M, et al. The psychosis high-risk state: a comprehensive state-of-the-art review. JAMA psychiatry 2013 70, (1):107-120. DOI: 10.1001/jamapsychiatry.2013.269

[62] Kebir O, Chaumette B, Rivollier F, Miozzo F, Perreault LL, Barhdadi A, Provost S, Plaze M, Bourgin J, Gaillard R, Mezger V. Methylomic changes during conversion to psychosis. Molecular psychiatry. 2017 Apr;22(4):512-518. DOI: 10.1038/mp.2016.53

[63] Bang M, Kang JI, Kim SJ, Park JY, Kim KR, Lee SY, Park K, Lee E, Lee SK, An SK. Reduced DNA Methylation of the Oxytocin Receptor Gene Is Associated With Anhedonia-Asociality in Women With Recent-Onset Schizophrenia and Ultra-high Risk for Psychosis. Schizophrenia Bulletin. 2019 Oct 24;45(6):1279-1290. DOI: 10.1093/schbul/sbz016.

[64] Popovic D, Schmitt A, Kaurani L, Senner F, Papiol S, Malchow B, Fischer A, Schulze TG, Koutsouleris N, Falkai P. Childhood trauma in schizophrenia: current findings and research perspectives. Frontiers in neuroscience. 2019 Mar 21;13:274. DOI: 10.3389/fnins.2019.00274

[65] Fachim HA, Loureiro CM, Corsi-Zuelli F, Shuhama R, Louzada-Junior P, Menezes PR, Dalton CF, Del-Ben CM, Reynolds GP.

GRIN2B promoter methylation deficits in early-onset schizophrenia and its association with cognitive function. Epigenomics. 2019 Mar;11(4):401-410. DOI: 10.2217/epi-2018-0127

[66] Mak M, Samochowiec J, Frydecka D, Pełka-Wysiecka J, Szmida E, Karpiński P, Sąsiadek MM, Piotrowski P, Samochowiec A, Misiak B. First-episode schizophrenia is associated with a reduction of HERV-K methylation in peripheral blood. Psychiatry research. 2019 Jan 1;271:459-463. DOI: 10.1016/j.psychres.2018.12.012

[67] Gulchina Y, Xu SJ, Snyder MA, Elefant F, Gao WJ. Epigenetic mechanisms underlying NMDA receptor hypofunction in the prefrontal cortex of juvenile animals in the MAM model for schizophrenia. Journal of neurochemistry. 2017 Nov;143(3):320-333. DOI: 10.1111/jnc.14101

[68] Montano C, Taub MA, Jaffe A, Briem E, Feinberg JI, Trygvadottir R, Idrizi A, Runarsson A, Berndsen B, Gur RC, Moore TM. Association of DNA methylation differences with schizophrenia in an epigenome-wide association study. JAMA psychiatry. 2016 May 1;73(5):506-514. DOI: 10.1001/jamapsychiatry.2016.0144

[69] Pai S, Li P, Killinger B, Marshall L, Jia P, Liao J, Petronis A, Szabó PE, Labrie V. Differential methylation of enhancer at IGF2 is associated with abnormal dopamine synthesis in major psychosis. Nature communications. 2019 May 3;10(1):1-2. DOI: 10.1038/s41467-019-09786-7

[70] Walton E, Cecil CA, Suderman M, Liu J, Turner JA, Calhoun V, Ehrlich S, Relton CL, Barker ED. Longitudinal epigenetic predictors of amygdala: hippocampus volume ratio. Journal of Child Psychology and Psychiatry. 2017 Dec;58(12):1341-1350. DOI: 10.1111/jcpp.12740

[71] Bosch C, Muhaisen A, Pujadas L, Soriano E, Martínez A. Reelin exerts structural, biochemical and transcriptional regulation over presynaptic and postsynaptic elements in the adult hippocampus. Frontiers in cellular neuroscience. 2016 May 30;10:138. DOI: 10.3389/fncel.2016.00138

[72] Guidotti A, Grayson DR, Caruncho HJ. Epigenetic RELN dysfunction in schizophrenia and related neuropsychiatric disorders. Frontiers in cellular neuroscience. 2016 Apr 5;10:89. DOI: 10.3389/fncel.2016.00089

[73] Ho NF, Li Z, Ji F, Wang M, Kuswanto CN, Sum MY, Tng HY, Sitoh YY, Sim K, Zhou J. Hemispheric lateralization abnormalities of the white matter microstructure in patients with schizophrenia and bipolar disorder. Journal of Psychiatry & Neuroscience: JPN. 2017 Jul;42(4):242. DOI: 10.1503/jpn.160090

[74] DeRamus TP, Silva RF, Iraji A, Damaraju E, Belger A, Ford JM, McEwen SC, Mathalon DH, Mueller BA, Pearlson GD, Potkin SG. Covarying structural alterations in laterality of the temporal lobe in schizophrenia: A case for source-based laterality. NMR in Biomedicine. 2020 Jun;33(6):e4294. DOI: 10.1002/nbm.4294

[75] He H, Luo C, Li N, Li Z, Duan M, Yao G, Wang H, He M, Yao D. Altered asymmetries of diffusion and volumetry in basal ganglia of schizophrenia. Brain Imaging and Behavior. 2020 Jul 23:1-6. DOI: 10.1007/s11682-020-00286-7

[76] Abdolmaleky HM, Gower AC, Wong CK, Cox JW, Zhang X, Thiagalingam A, Shafa R, Sivaraman V, Zhou JR, Thiagalingam S. Aberrant transcriptomes and DNA methylomes define pathways that drive pathogenesis and loss of brain laterality/asymmetry in schizophrenia and bipolar disorder.

American Journal of Medical Genetics Part B: Neuropsychiatric Genetics. 2019 Mar;180(2):138-149. DOI: 10.1002/ajmg.b.32691

[77] Sempere LF, Freemantle S, Pitha-Rowe I, Moss E, Dmitrovsky E, Ambros V. Expression profiling of mammalian microRNAs uncovers a subset of brain-expressed microRNAs with possible roles in murine and human neuronal differentiation. Genome biology. 2004 Feb 1;5(3):R13. DOI: 10.1186/gb-2004-5-3-r13

[78] Huang W, Li MD. Differential allelic expression of dopamine D1 receptor gene (DRD1) is modulated by microRNA miR-504. Biological psychiatry. 2009 65 (8):702-705. DOI: 10.1016/j.biopsych.2008.11.024

[79] Huang T, Liu Y, Huang M, Zhao X, Cheng L. Wnt1-cre-mediated conditional loss of Dicer results in malformation of the midbrain and cerebellum and failure of neural crest and dopaminergic differentiation in mice. Journal of molecular cell biology. 2010 2 (3):152-163. DOI: 10.1093/jmcb/mjq008

[80] Rubin LH, Connelly JJ, Reilly JL, Carter CS, Drogos LL, Pournajafi-Nazarloo H, Ruocco AC, Keedy SK, Matthew I, Tandon N, Pearlson GD. Sex and diagnosis-specific associations between DNA methylation of the oxytocin receptor gene with emotion processing and temporal-limbic and prefrontal brain volumes in psychotic disorders. Biological Psychiatry: Cognitive Neuroscience and Neuroimaging. 2016 Mar 1;1(2):141-151. DOI: 10.1016/j.bpsc.2015.10.003

[81] Garcia-Ruiz B, Moreno L, Muntané G, Sánchez-Gistau V, Gutiérrez-Zotes A, Martorell L, Labad J, Vilella E. Leukocyte and brain DDR1 hypermethylation is altered in psychosis and is correlated with stress and inflammatory markers. Epigenomics. 2020 Feb;12(3):251-265. DOI: 10.2217/epi-2019-0191

[82] Fachim HA, Srisawat U, Dalton CF, Reynolds GP. Parvalbumin promoter hypermethylation in postmortem brain in schizophrenia. Epigenomics. 2018 May;10(5):519-524. DOI: 10.2217/epi-2017-0159

[83] de Castro-Catala M, van Nierop M, Barrantes-Vidal N, Cristóbal-Narváez P, Sheinbaum T, Kwapil TR, Peña E, Jacobs N, Derom C, Thiery E, van Os J. Childhood trauma, BDNF Val66Met and subclinical psychotic experiences. Attempt at replication in two independent samples. Journal of psychiatric research. 2016 Dec 1;83: 121-129. DOI: 10.1016/j.jpsychires.2016.08.014

[84] Ikegame T, Bundo M, Okada N, Murata Y, Koike S, Sugawara H, Saito T, Ikeda M, Owada K, Fukunaga M, Yamashita F. Promoter activity-based case-control association study on SLC6A4 highlighting hypermethylation and altered amygdala volume in male patients with schizophrenia. bioRxiv. 2020 Jan 1. DOI: 10.1093/schbul/sbaa075

[85] Gilbert TM, Zürcher NR, Wu CJ, Bhanot A, Hightower BG, Kim M, Albrecht DS, Wey HY, Schroeder FA, Rodriguez-Thompson A, Morin TM. PET neuroimaging reveals histone deacetylase dysregulation in schizophrenia. The Journal of clinical investigation. 2019 Jan 2;129(1):364-372. DOI: 10.1172/JCI123743

[86] Schroeder FA, Gilbert TM, Feng N, Taillon BD, Volkow ND, Innis RB, Hooker JM, Lipska BK. Expression of HDAC2 but not HDAC1 transcript is reduced in dorsolateral prefrontal cortex of patients with schizophrenia. ACS chemical neuroscience. 2017 Mar 15;8(3):662-668. DOI: 10.1021/acschemneuro.6b00372

[87] Rivollier F, Chaumette B, Bendjemaa N, Chayet M, Millet B, Jaafari N, Barhdadi A, Lemieux Perreault LP, Provost S, Dubé MP, Gaillard R. Methylomic changes in individuals with psychosis, prenatally exposed to endocrine disrupting compounds: Lessons from diethylstilbestrol. PloS one. 2017 Apr 13;12(4):e0174783. DOI: 10.1371/journal.pone.0174783

[88] Rusconi F, Battaglioli E, Venturin M. Psychiatric Disorders and lncRNAs: A Synaptic Match. International Journal of Molecular Sciences. 2020 Jan;21(9):3030. DOI: 10.3390/ijms21093030

[89] Punzi G, Bharadwaj R, Ursini G. Neuroepigenetics of schizophrenia. InProgress in molecular biology and translational science 2018 Jan 1 (Vol. 158, pp. 195-226). Academic Press. DOI: 10.1016/bs.pmbts.2018.04.010

[90] NUMACHI Y, YOSHIDA S, YAMASHITA M, FUJIYAMA K, NAKA M, MATSUOKA H, SATO M, SORA I. Psychostimulant alters expression of DNA methyltransferase mRNA in the rat brain. Annals of the New York Academy of Sciences. 2004 Oct;1025(1):102-109. DOI: 10.1196/annals.1316.013

[91] Nohesara S, Ghadirivasfi M, Barati M, Ghasemzadeh MR, Narimani S, Mousavi-Behbahani Z, Joghataei M, Soleimani M, Taban M, Mehrabi S, Thiagalingam S. Methamphetamine-induced psychosis is associated with DNA hypomethylation and increased expression of AKT1 and key dopaminergic genes. American Journal of Medical Genetics Part B: Neuropsychiatric Genetics. 2016 Dec;171(8):1180-1189. DOI: 10.1002/ajmg.b.32506

[92] Jourdon A, Scuderi S, Capauto D, Abyzov A, Vaccarino FM. PsychENCODE and beyond: transcriptomics and epigenomics of brain development and organoids. Neuropsychopharmacology. 2021 Jan;46(1):70-85. DOI: 10.1038/s41386-020-0763-3

[93] Kubota T, Miyake K, Hariya N, Mochizuki K. Epigenetics as a basis for diagnosis of neurodevelopmental disorders: challenges and opportunities. Expert review of molecular diagnostics. 2014 Jul 1;14(6):685-697. DOI: 10.1586/14737159.2014.925805

[94] Kular L, Kular S. Epigenetics applied to psychiatry: clinical opportunities and future challenges. Psychiatry and clinical neurosciences. 2018 Apr;72(4):195-211. DOI: 10.1111/pcn.12634

[95] Peedicayil J. Epigenetic biomarkers in psychiatric disorders. British journal of pharmacology. 2008 Nov;155(6):795-796. DOI: 10.1038/bjp.2008.254

[96] Melas PA, Rogdaki M, Ösby U, Schalling M, Lavebratt C, Ekström TJ. Epigenetic aberrations in leukocytes of patients with schizophrenia: association of global DNA methylation with antipsychotic drug treatment and disease onset. The FASEB Journal. 2012 Jun;26(6):2712-2718. DOI: 10.1096/fj.11-202069

[97] Walton E, Cecil CA, Suderman M, Liu J, Turner JA, Calhoun V, Ehrlich S, Relton CL, Barker ED. Longitudinal epigenetic predictors of amygdala: hippocampus volume ratio. Journal of Child Psychology and Psychiatry. 2017 Dec;58(12):1341-1350. DOI: 10.1111/jcpp.12740

Chapter 7

DNA Methyltransferases and Schizophrenia: Current Status

Pranay Amruth Maroju and Kommu Naga Mohan

Abstract

Schizophrenia (SZ) is a complex disorder without a single cause but with multiple etiologies. Monozygotic twin studies suggesting high discordant rates provide evidence for epigenetic mechanisms among the factors that result in increased susceptibility. Among the different epigenetic modifications in mammals, DNA methylation mediated by DNA methyltransferases (DNMTs) is the most-well studied. Studies on post-mortem brain samples and blood samples of SZ patients revealed altered levels of most DNMTs. In addition, some recent studies also reported disease-associated SNPs in the DNMT genes. While the effects of dysregulation of DNMTs are beginning to be understood, many unanswered questions remain. Here, we review the current evidences that shed light on the relationship between DNMT dysregulation and SZ, and suggest the possible strategies to address some of the unanswered questions.

Keywords: Schizophrenia, DNA methyltransferases, DNA methylation, Dysregulation, Abnormal neurogenesis

1. Introduction

Schizophrenia (SZ) is a severe and chronic mental disorder with an incidence of ~1%, affecting ~20 million people worldwide [1]. The main symptoms of SZ include hallucination, delusion, abnormal disorganized behavior, disorganized speech, disturbances of emotions such as marked apathy, etc. The disorder is associated with considerable disability and can affect educational and occupational performance with 2–3 times increased likelihood of death earlier than the general population [2].

SZ is a complex disorder with no single causative factor but with multiple etiologies (**Table 1**). The five main factors that are believed to result in increased risk are: physical and chemical changes in brain [3], pregnancy or birth complications [4], childhood trauma [5], genetic [6] -and epigenetic [8]. Among these, a high risk among first-degree relatives compared to the general population and increased risk in monozygotic than dizygotic twins suggest genetic factors [7]. However, the observed concordance rates (~50%) in monozygotic twins that were much lesser than expected for a purely genetic risk (nearly 100%) suggest the contribution of epigenetic mechanisms to SZ [9].

Recent data based on brain imaging and molecular-genetic studies suggest that SZ is a form of neurodevelopmental disorder [10]. The neurodevelopmental hypothesis for SZ suggests pathological neurodevelopment during first and second

IntechOpen

S. No	Factor	Comment	References
1	Physical and chemical changes in brain.	Subtle structural changes have been observed in post-mortem brain samples of SZ patients. Imbalances in neurotransmitters such as dopamine and glutamate have been linked to SZ.	[3]
2	Pregnancy or birth complications	Low birth weight, infection during pregnancy, asphyxia, premature labour, maternal obesity diagnosis in pregnancy, etc. have been associated with SZ in the offspring.	[4]
3	Childhood trauma	There is an increased risk to experience SZ if there is death or permanent separation of one or both parents.	[5]
4	Genetic	The risk in identical twins (1 in 2) is four times higher than non-identical twins (1 in 8). These risks are much higher than for general population (1 in 100).	[6, 7]
5	Epigenetic	Monozygotic twins show only 45–50% concordance.	[8, 9]

Table 1.
Risk factors for schizophrenia.

trimesters of pregnancy results in altered neuronal circuits which in turn result in psychosis in adolescents or young adults when exposed to increased biological or psychological stress. Evidences in support of this hypothesis comes from genetic studies that identified affected genes and risk factors during perinatal life that may disrupt the normal process of neurodevelopment. In addition, studies over the past 20 years showed that in comparison with controls, SZ patients after the onset exhibit accelerated aging-related loss of brain tissue [11]. Specifically, the patients show increased age-related reduction in the proportion of grey matter compared with controls [12]. These findings suggest that altered neurodevelopment may underlie the processes associated with SZ.

2. Epigenetic mechanisms

As mentioned above, evidence on the contribution of epigenetic mechanisms in SZ comes from monozygotic twin studies wherein the concordance rates are only ~50%. This low concordance rate suggests the interplay of genes and environment resulting in SZ. Because of this interplay, the epigenetic mechanisms have been suggested to be among the etiological factors [8]. Epigenetic mechanisms are defined as processes that can alter the patterns of gene expression without causing a change in the DNA sequence [13]. These mechanisms operate at the levels of transcription, mRNA stability and translation (**Table 2**). At the level of transcription, mammalian genes can be regulated by covalent modifications of the DNA [19], modifications of N-terminal tails of histones [15], microRNAs [20], circular RNAs [17] and long noncoding RNAs [21]. A number of modifications of RNA have been reported to influence mRNA stability and efficiency of translation. These modifications and their roles are described elsewhere [22, 23]. Because of epigenetic differences, genetically identical cells in a multicellular organism express different sets of genes that confer cell type – specific identity and function [24]. The most well studied epigenetic modification is methylation of the 5th carbon in the cytosine residues in the genomic DNA, often referred to as cytosine methylation. This modification mostly occurs in the CpG dinucleotides because of the maintenance mechanism in a post-replicative manner involving hemi-methylated DNA [see below]. As such, DNA methylation is often used as a synonym to CpG methylation

Mechanisms	Machinery	Comment
1. DNA Methylation 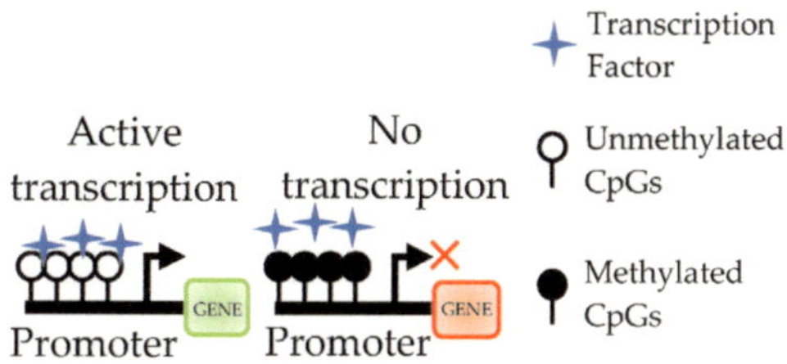	Establishment and maintenance: DNMTs Erasure: TETs, AID/APOBECs.	Altered methylation patterns and gene expression patterns observed in SZ [14].
2. Histone tail modifications 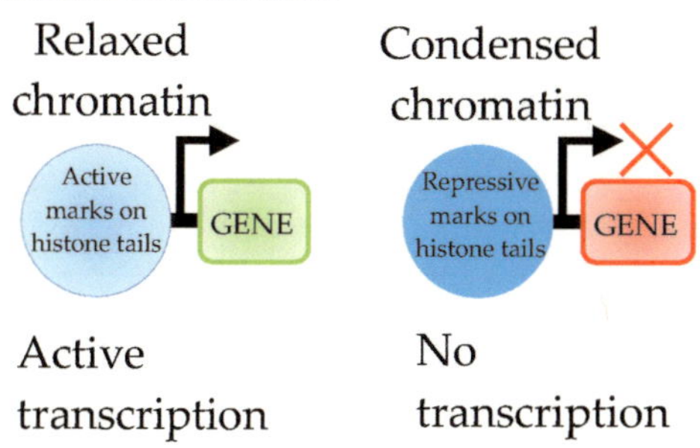	Establishment: HATs, HMTs Erasure: HDMs and HDACs.	Aberrant histone modifications were reported in SZ [15].
3. MicroRNAs 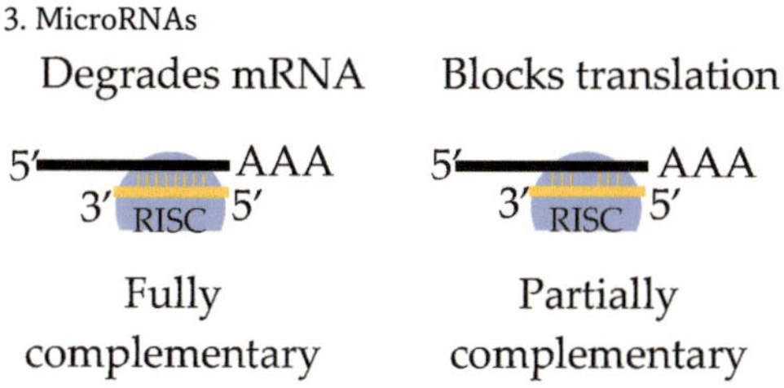	DROSHA, EXPORTIN, DICER, RISC and ARGONAUTE	Altered miRNA profiles were reported in SZ [16].
4. Circular RNAs 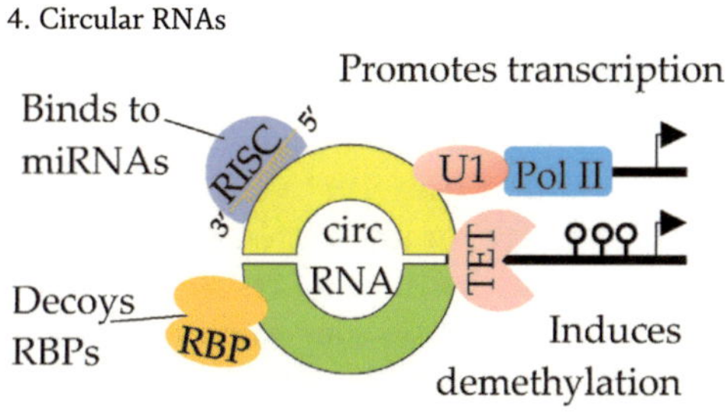	RNA binding proteins, muscleblind (MBL), quaking and adenosine deaminase.	Multiple circRNAs have been confirmed to play important roles in the occurrence and development of SZ [17].
5. Long non-coding RNAs 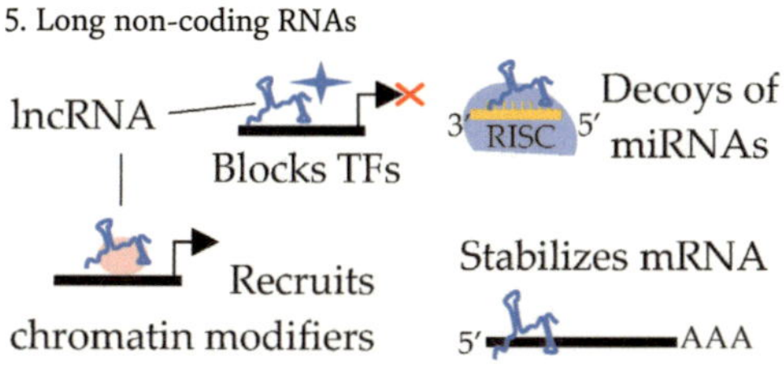	PRC1: Polycomb Repressive Group proteins.	Long non-coding RNAs are associated with SZ and effects in the neuronal structure [18].

Table 2.
Epigenetic mechanisms in regulating gene expression.

in mammals. A family of enzymes, referred to as DNA methyltransferases (DNMTs) are responsible for establishment and maintenance of DNA methylation [25]. Several studies that focused on the relationship between DNA methylation and gene expression showed an inverse correlation, meaning that DNA methylation is often associated with repressed state of the promoters [26]. In case of histones, the lysines in the N-terminal tails of core histones can either be acetylated or methylated. These modifications occur on the same lysine residues and are therefore mutually exclusive [27]. Whereas histone lysine acetylation is always associated with gene expression, histone methylation is associated with either expression or silencing depending on the residues involved [28]. For example, methylation at lysine 9 of histone H3 (H3-K9) or H3-K27 is associated with silencing. On the other hand, H3-K4 or H3-K36 methylation is associated with gene expression. Histone methyltransferases and histone acetyltransferases are two families of enzymes for imparting the two covalent modifications of the N-terminal tails of the core histones [29]. As in case of DNA methylation, histone marks are also heritable. The covalently modified nucleosomes from the parental chromatin are segregated equally among the two daughter DNA molecules so that additional nucleosomes containing histone marks identical to the parental nucleosomes are assembled [30]. Both DNA methylation and histone modifications are reversible involving different categories of enzymes and processes. The machinery of DNA methylation and demethylation is described in the next section [Section 2.1]. With regard to the histone modifications, histone demethylases (HDMs), histone methyltransferases (HMTs), histone acetyltransferases (HATs) and histone deacetylases (HDACs) together play a role in erasure and establishment of histone modification marks [31]. HDMs remove methyl groups from the lysines of the core histones so that the unmethylated lysines can be acetylated by HATs. HDACs, on the other hand, remove acetyl groups from the acetylated lysines so that the same residues can be methylated by HMTs.

Apart from covalent modifications of the genome, long noncoding RNAs (lnc RNAs), microRNAs (miRNAs) and circular RNAs (circRNAs) also play an important role in regulating gene expression. Of these, circRNAs and miRNAs regulate expression at post-transcriptional levels whereas lncRNAs can regulate at both transcriptional and post-transcriptional levels. Lnc RNAs are ≥200 nucleotides, do not encode any protein and regulate genes at the both transcriptional and post-transcriptional levels [32]. At the level of transcription, lncRNAs either can promote histone modifications and chromatin condensation or recruit transcription factors to facilitate gene expression or evict transcription factors and result in gene repression. In addition, lncRNAs are also known to influence alternative splicing, polysome recruitment to enable translation, act as decoys for microRNAs (miRNAs) and regulate mRNA stability. The miRNAs, on the other hand cause translational repression of the target mRNAs. Each miRNA is ~22 bases long and can recognize multiple targets having a few mismatches at their 3′-ends [33]. In cases, where there is no mismatch, miRNA can induce degradation of the target mRNA sequence [34]. CircRNAs are generated by back-splicing or non-colinear splicing of pre-mRNA molecules and may include both exonic and intronic sequences [35]. In addition to competing with canonical splicing and controlling the levels of the corresponding protein-coding mRNAs, circRNAs can also act as protein decoys or miRNA sponges to regulate gene expression [36].

2.1 DNA methylation and demethylation machinery

Of the different epigenetic mechanisms influencing gene expression described above, DNA methylation-mediated regulation of gene expression is the most-well studied. DNA methylation is established and maintained by DNMT family of enzymes whereas different mechanisms exist for demethylation (**Figure 1A**). Of the four members of DNMTs that facilitate DNA methylation, DNMT3L does not have an active methyltransferase (catalytic) domain. DNMT3A and 3B are *de novo* methyltransferases of which DNMT3A is mainly responsible for establishment of

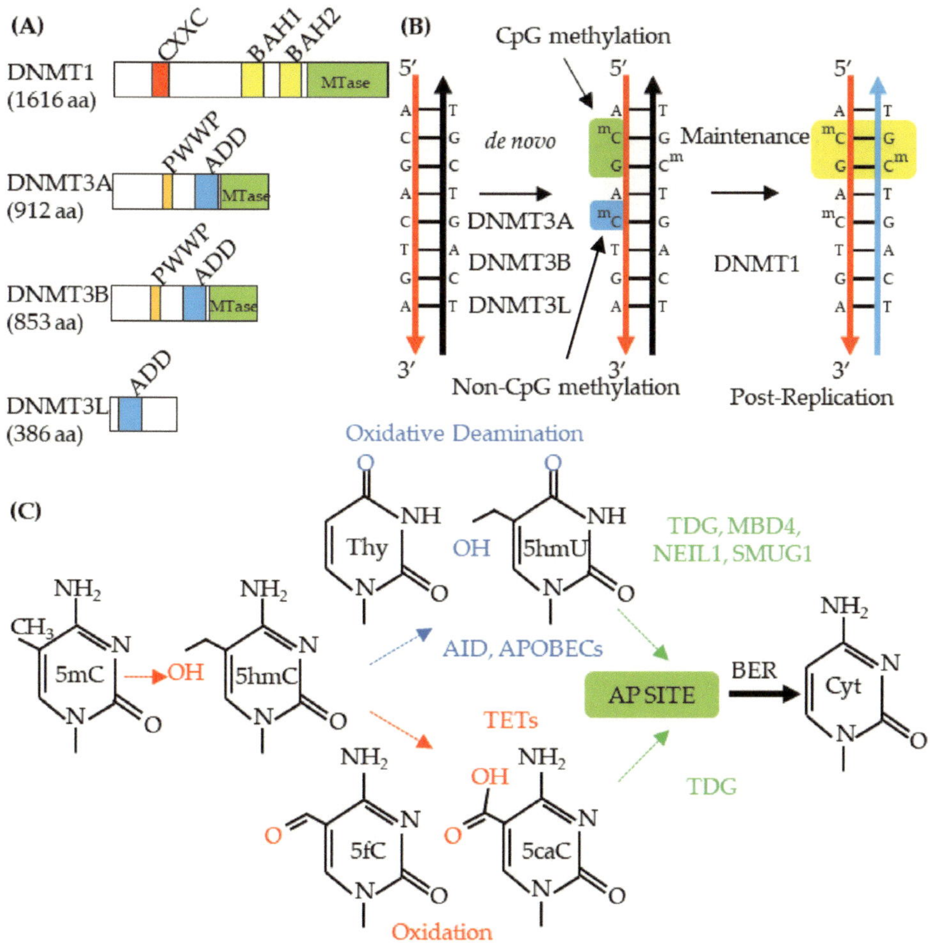

Figure 1.
DNA methylation and demethylation machinery. (A) Domains of DNMTs. CXXC: Cys-X-X-Cys domain, BAH: Bromo-Adjacent Homology domain, MTase: Methyltransferase domain, PWWP: Pro-Trp-Trp-Pro domain, ADD: ATRX-DNMT3-DNMT3L domain (B) Cytosines are methylated by de novo *methyltransferases DNMT3A and DNMT3B with the help of DNMT3L. Only methylated CpGs are maintained by DNMT1. (C) Different pathways of demethylation of methylated cytosines (5mC). TET: ten-eleven translocation (TET) proteins, AID/APOBEC: activity-induced cytidine deaminase/ apolipoprotein B mRNA editing complex, Thy: thymine. TDG: Thymine-DNA glycosylase, AP: apurinic/apyrimidinic site, BER: base-excision repair. 5hmU: 5-hydroxymethyluracil, 5hmC: 5-hydroxymethylcytosine, 5fC: 5-formylcytosine and 5caC: 5-carboxylcytosine.*

methylation in imprinted genes whereas DNMT3B establishes methylation in pericentric repetitive regions [37]. DNMT1 is a maintenance methyltransferase, which methylates the daughter DNA strand in the hemi-methylated DNA generated after replication (**Figure 1B**). In this process, the methylated CpG sites in the parental strands serve as information to methylate the complementary CpG sites in the daughter strand. Demethylation, on the other hand can be achieved by cytidine deaminases or Ten-Eleven Translocation (TET) enzymes [38] (**Figure 1C**). Cytidine deaminases such as activated induced cytidine deaminase (AID) and apolipoprotein B mRNA editing enzyme catalytic polypeptide 1 (APOBEC1) catalyze the conversion of methylcytosine to thymine [39], leading to T:G mismatches. These mismatches are repaired by base excision repair machinery that incorporates unmodified cytosine. The TET enzymes hydroxymethylate the methylated cytosines which are further processed into oxidized forms of cytosine (5-formylcytosine and 5-carboxycytosine) that are further subjected to base excision repair resulting in active demethylation. Hydroxymethylcytosine results in passive demethylation via DNA replication because of absence of methylgroup in the parental strand in the hemimethylated DNA.

2.2 DNA methylation studies in schizophrenia

Initial studies on DNA methylation differences between SZ patients and controls, and among discordant monozygotic twins focused on candidate genes identified by genetic studies. For example, Abdolmaleky et al. [40] by using DNA from frontal lobes of post-mortem brain samples showed ~50% increased methylation in the RELN promoter. Subsequent DNA methylation studies focused on genes involved in Dopaminergic [41], GABAergic [42], Glutamatergic [43], serotonergic pathways [44] of neurotransmission and genes such as BDNF [45]. These studies used DNAs either post-mortem brain samples or peripheral blood lymphocytes. However, the data did not always yield consistent reports. For example, in case of BDNF promoter IV, decreased DNA methylation was observed in peripheral blood in a study by Kordi et al. [46] whereas, Ikegame et al. [47] and Ümit Sertan Çöpoğlu et al. [48] reported no change in the methylation levels in the same tissue. Subsequent studies which used genome-wide methylation analysis identified many genes showing statistically significant differences in DNA methylation, but the effective values or the degree of methylation differences observed were not large enough to demonstrate a biological effect such as altered expression. For example, in one of the first studies, Mill et al. [49] by using microarrays identified genes RPL39 and WDR18 with increased methylation in the promoter upstream regions of 8% and 3%, respectively. Studies conducted after these observations used a variety of technologies such as Methylated DNA Immunoprecipitation (MeDIP) – sequencing and Illumina-27 K and 450 K arrays and reported differentially methylated sequences with low effective values. Importantly these studies identified genes with little or no overlap among the top gene hits corresponding to the most significant differentially methylated sites [50]. Nevertheless, some of these genome-wide studies also identified methylation differences in candidate genes such as COMT [51], GAD1, RELN [52] and BDNF [53]. Although these genome-wide studies did not yield common genes with significant differences in DNA methylation, bioinformatic analyses revealed common pathways. For example, methylome data using the blood DNAs revealed the involvement of functioning of the immune system [54]. This in turn is in agreement with the genome-wide association studies that identified immune-related genes including the major histocompatibility locus [55]. Another common pathway identified in both blood– and DNA- based studies is the neurodevelopmental processes [56]. The DNA methylation studies were also extended to study the effects on gene expression. In one such study, Liu *et al.* [57] identified 16 differentially methylated sites using a case–control approach. When the corresponding 16 genes were studied only five genes showed an inverse correlation of expression with methylation whereas two showed a positive correlation. The remaining genes showed no difference in the level of expression. Besides analysis of gene-related regions of the genome, bulk DNA methylation in SZ patients was also investigated. In such studies, Bonsch *et al.* [58] observed lower levels of methylation in peripheral blood monocytes of patients among discordant monozygotic twins. Meals *et al.* [59] also found a decreased global methylation levels in leukocytes of patients compared to normal individuals. However, these studies are not in agreement with Bromberg *et al.* [60] who did not observe any difference in the global methylation levels in leukocytes. Overall studies on the global methylation levels were inconclusive and likely to be influenced by factors such as age, gender, medication and smoking behavior. In summary, some but not all studies observed significant differences in DNA methylation levels in the candidate genes whereas genome-wide studies indicated the involvement of neurodevelopmental processes and immune system function. These results are consistent with the model of etiology that SZ is a complex disorder with no single causative factor.

2.3 Dysregulated DNMTs in schizophrenia

Epigenetic processes and epigenetic modifications are tightly controlled to enable normal mammalian development. In this context, the presence of aberrant DNA methylation patterns affecting the candidate genes suggests the possibility of the role of dysregulation of epigenetic machinery in SZ. Investigations on dysregulation of DNA methylation machinery in SZ dates back to 2005 when Veldic *et al.* [61] reported increased DNMT1 levels in the GABAergic interneurons of post-mortem brain tissues of SZ patients. This increase was also correlated with increased promoter methylation and decreased expression of *REELIN,* an extracellular matrix protein and *GAD67*, an enzyme involved in production of GABA. Importantly, DNMT1 inhibitors were reported to decrease hypermethylation and increased expression of the two genes [62]. Subsequently, HDAC inhibitors were also shown to relieve the repression associated with DNMT1 overexpression to an extent similar to DNMT1 inhibitors [63]. These results suggest the potential of epigenetic drugs in ameliorating the phenotypes associated with SZ. Later experiments in brain tissues of patients revealed that at increased levels, DNMT1 binds to *REELIN*, *GAD67* and *BDNF* promoters in cortex but not cerebellum. Further, this selective cortex-specific binding is not associated with any changes in the levels of DNA methylation [64]. The authors suggested that increased DNMT1-associated downregulation of the three genes can be independent of the catalytic activity of DNMT1. As mentioned above, DNMT1 is a maintenance methyltransferase and cannot introduce new methyl groups in the DNA. Therefore, hypermethylation of *REELIN* and *GAD67* is possible only if there is *de novo* methylation followed by maintenance methylation of DNMT1. Not surprisingly, overexpression of DNMT1 as well as DNMT3A was subsequently observed in post-mortem brain samples as well as peripheral blood lymphocytes of SZ patients [65]. Further, DNMT3B overexpression was also reported in peripheral blood lymphocytes but is not reported as of date in post-mortem brain tissues of SZ patients. Since both DNMT3A and 3B are required for *de novo* methylation, it is not unexpected that DNMT3B would also be overexpressed in the brain tissues of the patients. In addition to human studies, experiments using offspring of prenatal restrained stressed mice also confirmed the association of increased DNMTs with SZ-associated phenotypes. In the progeny, DNMT1 and 3A protein levels were high with increased binding of DNMT1 and MeCP2 (Methyl-CpG binding protein 2) and repression of *REELIN* and *GAD67* promoters [66].

Taken together, there is reasonable argument for DNMT1 and DNMT3A and, possibly DNMT3B overexpression as risk factors for SZ. However, the information on the number of genes dysregulated due to DNMT1 overexpression was limited only three (*REELIN, GAD67* and *BDNF*). By taking DNMTs as risk-conferring genes, Saradalekshmi *et al.* [67] investigated whether any SNPs of DNMTs are associated with SZ. In this case–control study, minor alleles at rs2114724 and rs2228611 of *Dnmt1*, rs2424932 and rs1569686 of *Dnmt*3B and rs2070565 in *Dnmt3L* showed significant association with SZ. The authors also reported that rs2424932 showed an association in male patients whereas rs1569686 was associated with an earlier onset in patients with family history. Bioinformatic analysis on the effects of these SNPs suggested that the minor alleles affect the splicing of *Dnmt1* or *Dnmt3L* transcript or reduce the levels of expression of *Dnmt3B*. However, functional studies on these SNPs were not reported yet.

2.4 Models of dysregulated DNMTs

In the light of reports suggesting increased DNMT1 and/or DNMT3A levels as risk factors for SZ, it is important to understand the effects of their overexpression on neurodevelopment. Unfortunately, overexpression of DNMT1 results in mid-gestational lethality in mice [68] making it impossible to generate animal models with constitutive overexpression. In addition, reduction of DNMT1 protein levels, but not its absence, appears to be an essential step for differentiation [69]. In this context, it is also difficult to generate mice conditional alleles of *Dnmt1* that enable neurogenesis-specific overexpression. Therefore, we proposed that cell-based models that either over express DNMT3A or DNMT1 or together serve as useful tools for studying the effects on neurogenesis. Specifically, embryonic stem cells (ESCs) are attractive because they provide opportunities to investigate the effects of DNMT1 and /or DNMT3A overexpression at different stages of neural differentiation. For instance, during the induction of neuronal differentiation, the ESCs are first differentiated into embryoid bodies (EBs) to obtain progenitor cells with ectoderm, endoderm and mesoderm specification. From EB stage, the cells can be differentiated into neuronal progenitor cells (NPCs) and subsequently into neurons.

In order to study the effects of DNMT1 overexpression on neurogenesis, D'Aiuto *et al.* [70] utilized *Dnmt1*$^{tet/tet}$ (*Tet/Tet*), a mouse embryonic stem cell line that overexpresses DNMT1 (**Figure 2A**). This cell line was generated by insertion of *tet-off* cassettes between the *Dnmt1* promoters and the start codons of both chromosomes [71]. As a result, the endogenous *Dnmt1* promoter expressed tTA, a transactivator that binds to the CMV-*tet operator* (*TetO + CMV* sequence present at the 3′-end of the *tet-off* cassettes. This resulted in increased expression of DNMT1 in the *Tet/Tet* ESCs. When doxycycline is added to this cell line, tTA became inactive and could not express *Dnmt1* and making the genome hypomethylated. When the *Tet/Tet* ESCs were used for neuronal differentiation by the authors, there was reduction in DNMT1 levels in embryoid bodies with no difference between the wild-type (*R1*) and *Tet/Tet* cells. However, neurons differentiated from the *Tet/Tet* cells showed abnormal dendritic branching (**Figure 2B**), increased activity of N-methyl-D-aspartate (NMDA) receptor (**Figure 2C**) and increased levels of the NR1 subunit of the receptor. In this study, the authors reported that increased DNMT1 levels did not result in any hypermethylation of *Reelin* or *Gad67* promoters. This finding was not surprising because DNMT1 was only a maintenance methyltransferase and new methylation marks are established only by the *de novo* methyltransferases. Although this study indicated that DNMT1 overexpression results in abnormal neurogenesis, the effects on the levels of SZ-associated gene transcripts, particularly on genes such as *Gad67*, *Reelin* and *Bdnf* were not investigated.

In a recent study, Saxena *et al.* [72] used a modified neuronal differentiation method that resulted in increased expression of DNMT1 in *Tet/Tet* neurons (**Figure 2D**). These results suggested that *Tet/Tet* neurons were suitable for studying the expression levels of SZ-associated genes in presence of increased DNMT1 levels [73]. When 15 SZ-associated genes were tested between the *Tet/Tet* and *R1* neurons, 13 showed significantly altered transcript levels of which, 11 showed identical patterns of dysregulation as in patients (**Figure 2E**). Eight of these 11 also showed significantly altered transcript levels in *Tet/Tet* ESCs but the patterns were similar to *Tet/Tet* neurons in only five cases. These results suggested that the dysregulation patterns of the SZ-associated genes varied during the stages of

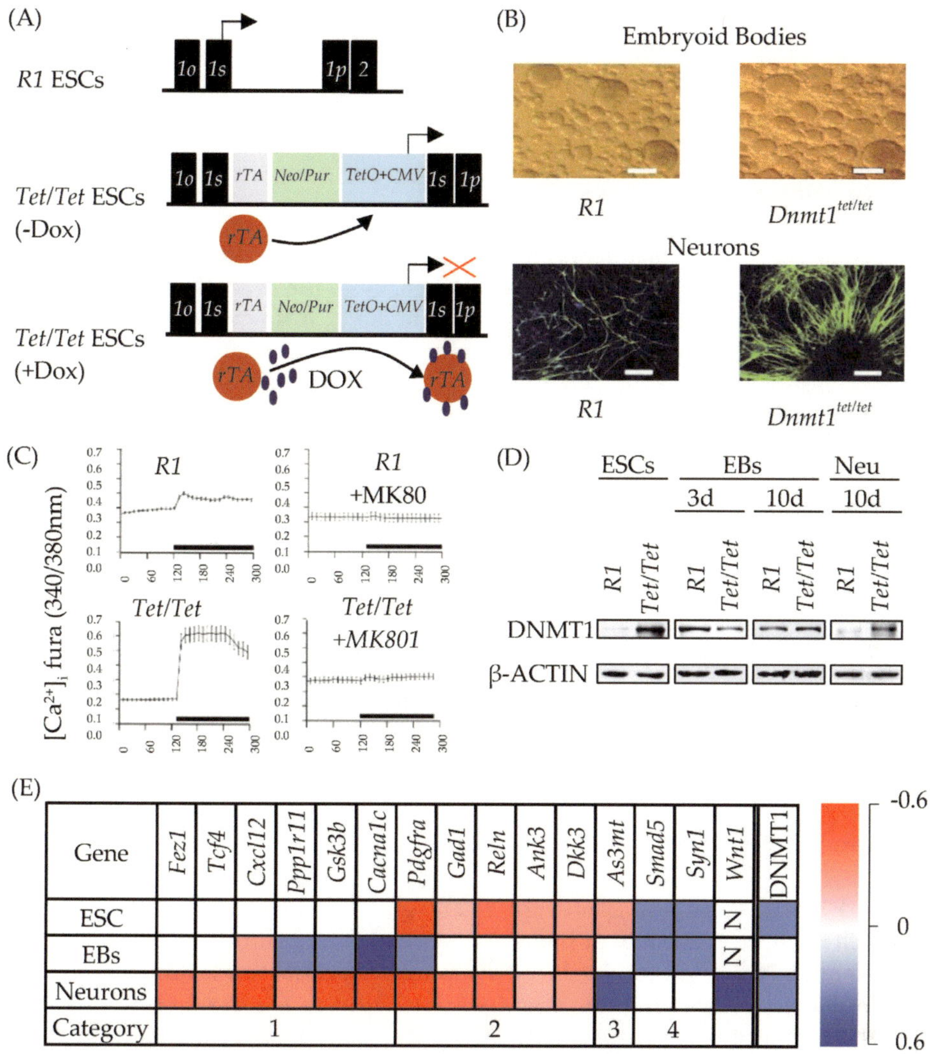

Figure 2.
(A) Generation of Tet/Tet *ESC line.* R1*: wild-type. Oocyte (1o), somatic cell (1s) and pachytene spermatocyte (1p) promoters are shown. (B) Embryoid bodies (EBs) and neurons differentiated from* R1 *and* Tet/Tet *ESCs. Neo/Pur: Neomycin and puromycin selection markers. (C) Increased NMDA receptor activity in* Tet/Tet *neurons. Compared to* R1 *neurons, when glutamate was added, the calcium uptake is higher in* Tet/Tet *neurons. This uptake is inhibited when MK801 (inhibitor of NMDA receptor) was used. (D) Western blot analysis of DNMT1 in* Tet/Tet *ESCs, EBs and neurons. (E) Four distinct categories of the 15 SZ-associated gene transcripts studied in* Tet/Tet *and* R1 *cells. Direction of change is indicated as per the color key. Red color indicates decreased transcript levels whereas increased transcript levels are shown in blue. Absence of color indicates no change.*

pluripotency and neuronal differentiation. The authors then used doxycycline to turn off *Dnmt1* and studied whether dysregulation observed in *Tet/Tet* ESCs could be reversed. Out of the eight genes tested in ESCs, the direction of transcript dysregulation for only four genes was reversed. These results suggested that by using DNMT1 inhibitors, it may not be possible to reverse DNMT1 overexpression-associated dysregulation of certain SZ-associated genes. Importantly, in this study, the authors did not observe any significant difference in the levels of methylation of the promoters of the affected genes either in ESCs or neurons. These results indicated that dysregulation of the genes studied in *Tet/Tet* neurons could be due to catalytic activity-independent effects of DNMT1. While the results on the *Tet/Tet* cells undoubtedly revealed the effects of DNMT1 overexpression on a wider set of SZ-associated genes, details on the global effects of increased DNMT1 levels at the transcriptome and methylome levels are still awaited.

3. Conclusions

In conclusion, molecular details that connect DNMT1 overexpression with abnormal neurogenesis are beginning to emerge. With the availability of genome-wide methylation and transcriptome analysis methods, it is now possible to investigate the effects of DNMT1 overexpression in post-mortem brain samples of SZ patients. However, this effort requires an understanding on the incidence of DNMT1 overexpression in these samples. Of particular interest is to compare the effects of overexpression of DNMT1 or DNMT3A or both during the process of neuronal differentiation and the nature of the altered transcript levels. Whether the genes affected are only related to SZ or other neuropsychiatric disorders or neurodevelopmental disorders is an important question that needs to be addressed. Such information is useful to explore the contribution of epigenetic mechanisms in a wider spectrum of neurological disorders. In addition, improvement in the methods for generating genetically modified ESCs, their differentiation into specific types of neurons and development of brain organoids should help advance our understanding of the relationship between dysregulation of DNA methyltransferases and neurodevelopmental disorders such as schizophrenia.

Acknowledgements

Work in KNM's laboratory is supported by grants from Science and Engineering Research Board, Department of Biotechnology and Birla Institute of Technology and Science Pilani. PAM received fellowship from a project funded by the Department of Biotechnology and later from Centre for Human Disease Research (BITS Pilani). KNM received OPERA award (BITS Pilani) and partial funding from the Centre for Human Disease Research.

Conflict of interest

The authors declare no conflicts of interest.

Author details

Pranay Amruth Maroju[1] and Kommu Naga Mohan[1,2*]

1 Department of Biological Sciences, BITS Pilani Hyderabad Campus, Hyderabad, India

2 Centre for Human Disease Research, BITS Pilani Hyderabad Campus, Hyderabad, India

*Address all correspondence to: mohankn@hyderabad.bits-pilani.ac.in

References

[1] GBD 2017 Disease and Injury Incidence and Prevalence Collaborators. Global, regional, and national incidence, prevalence, and years lived with disability for 354 diseases and injuries for 195 countries and territories, 1990-2017: a systematic analysis for the Global Burden of Disease Study 2017. Lancet. 2018;392(10159):1789-1858. DOI: 10.1016/S0140-6736(18)32279-7.

[2] Laursen TM, Nordentoft M, Mortensen PB. Excess early mortality in schizophrenia. Annual Review of Clinical Psychology. 2014;10:425-48. DOI: 10.1146/annurev-clinpsy-032813-153657.

[3] Chen F, Bertelsen AB, Holm IE, Nyengaard JR, Rosenberg R, Dorph-Petersen KA. Hippocampal volume and cell number in depression, schizophrenia, and suicide subjects. Brain Research. 2020;15;1727:146546. DOI: 10.1016/j.brainres.2019.146546.

[4] Stilo SA, Murray RM. Non-Genetic Factors in Schizophrenia. Current Psychiatry Reports. 2019;14;21(10):100. DOI: 10.1007/s11920-019-1091-3.

[5] Popovic D, Schmitt A, Kaurani L, Senner F, Papiol S, Malchow B, Fischer A, Schulze TG, Koutsouleris N, Falkai P. Childhood Trauma in Schizophrenia: Current Findings and Research Perspectives. Frontiers in Neuroscience. 2019;21;13:274. DOI: 10.3389/fnins.2019.00274.

[6] Cardno AG, O'Donovan MC, and Owen MJ. Genetic Risk Factors for Schizophrenia. International Journal of Mental Health. 2000;13-38. Accessed February 1, 2021. http://www.jstor.org/stable/41344944.

[7] Chou IJ, Kuo CF, Huang YS, Grainge MJ, Valdes AM, See LC, Yu KH, Luo SF, Huang LS, Tseng WY, Zhang W and Doherty M. Familial Aggregation and Heritability of Schizophrenia and Co-aggregation of Psychiatric Illnesses in Affected Families. Schizophrenia Bulletin. 2017;43(5), 1070–1078. DOI: 10.1093/schbul/sbw159.

[8] Smigielski L, Jagannath V, Rössler W, Walitza S, Grünblatt E. Epigenetic mechanisms in schizophrenia and other psychotic disorders: a systematic review of empirical human findings. Molecular Psychiatry. 2020;25(8):1718-1748. DOI: 10.1038/s41380-019-0601-3.

[9] Castillo-Fernandez JE, Spector TD, Bell JT. Epigenetics of discordant monozygotic twins: implications for disease. Genome Medicine. 2014;31; 6(7):60. DOI: 10.1186/s13073-014-0060-z.

[10] Owen MJ, O'Donovan MC, Thapar A, Craddock N. Neurodevelopmental hypothesis of schizophrenia. The British Journal of Psychiatry. 2011;198(3):173-5. DOI: 10.1192/bjp.bp.110.084384.

[11] Olabi B, Ellison-Wright I, McIntosh AM, Wood SJ, Bullmore E, Lawrie SM. Are there progressive brain changes in schizophrenia? A meta-analysis of structural magnetic resonance imaging studies. Biological Psychiatry. 2011;70(1):88-96. DOI: 10.1016/j.biopsych.2011.01.032.

[12] Vita A, De Peri L, Deste G, Sacchetti E. Progressive loss of cortical gray matter in schizophrenia: a meta-analysis and meta-regression of longitudinal MRI studies. Translational Psychiatry. 2012;2(11):e190. DOI: 10.1038/tp.2012.116.

[13] Berger SL, Kouzarides T, Shiekhattar R, Shilatifard A. An operational definition of epigenetics. Genes and Development. 2009;23(7): 781-3. DOI: 10.1101/gad.1787609.

[14] Grayson D, Guidotti A. The Dynamics of DNA Methylation in Schizophrenia and Related Psychiatric Disorders. Neuropsychopharmacology. 2013;38,138–166. DOI: 10.1038/npp.2012.125.

[15] Thomas EA. Histone Posttranslational Modifications in Schizophrenia. Advances in Experimental Medicine and Biology. 2017;978:237-254. DOI: 10.1007/978-3-319-53889-1_13.

[16] Hauberg ME, Roussos P, Grove J, Børglum AD, Mattheisen M. Analyzing the Role of MicroRNAs in Schizophrenia in the Context of Common Genetic Risk Variants. JAMA Psychiatry. 2016;73(4):369–377. DOI:10.1001/jamapsychiatry.2015.3018.

[17] Li Z, Liu S, Li X, Zhao W, Li J, Xu Y. Circular RNA in Schizophrenia and Depression. Frontiers in Psychiatry. 2020;7;11:392. DOI: 10.3389/fpsyt.2020.00392.

[18] Merelo V, Durand D, Lescallette AR, Vrana KE, Hong LE, Faghihi MA, Bellon A. Associating schizophrenia, long non-coding RNAs and neurostructural dynamics. Frontiers in Molecular Neuroscience. 2015;30;8:57. DOI: 10.3389/fnmol.2015.00057.

[19] Attwood JT, Yung RL, Richardson BC. DNA methylation and the regulation of gene transcription. Cellular and Molecular Life Sciences. 2002;59(2):241-57. DOI: 10.1007/s00018-002-8420-z.

[20] O'Brien J, Hayder H, Zayed Y, Peng C. Overview of MicroRNA Biogenesis, Mechanisms of Actions, and Circulation. Frontiers in Endocrinology. 2018;3;9:402. DOI: 10.3389/fendo.2018.00402.

[21] Vance KW, Ponting CP. Transcriptional regulatory functions of nuclear long noncoding RNAs. Trends in Genetics. 2014;30(8):348-55. DOI: 10.1016/j.tig.2014.06.001.

[22] Boo SH, Kim YK. The emerging role of RNA modifications in the regulation of mRNA stability. Experimental and Molecular Medicine. 2020;52(3):400-408. DOI: 10.1038/s12276-020-0407-z.

[23] Wang X, Zhao BS, Roundtree IA, Lu Z, Han D, Ma H, Weng X, Chen K, Shi H, He C. N(6)-methyladenosine Modulates Messenger RNA Translation Efficiency. Cell. 2015;4;161(6):1388-99. DOI: 10.1016/j.cell.2015.05.014.

[24] Barrero MJ, Boué S, Izpisúa Belmonte JC. Epigenetic mechanisms that regulate cell identity. Cell Stem Cell. 2010;5;7(5):565-70. DOI: 10.1016/j.stem.2010.10.009.

[25] Chen T, Li E. Establishment and maintenance of DNA methylation patterns in mammals. Current Topics in Microbiology and Immunology. 2006;301:179-201. DOI: 10.1007/3-540-31390-7_6.

[26] Jones PA. Functions of DNA methylation: islands, start sites, gene bodies and beyond. Nature Review Genetics. 2012;29;13(7):484-92. DOI: 10.1038/nrg3230. PMID: 22641018.

[27] Nakayama J, Rice JC, Strahl BD, Allis CD, Grewal SI. Role of histone H3 lysine 9 methylation in epigenetic control of heterochromatin assembly. Science. 2001;6;292(5514):110-3. DOI: 10.1126/science.

[28] Peterson CL, Laniel MA. Histones and histone modifications. Current Biology. 2004;27;14(14):R546-51. DOI: 10.1016/j.cub.2004.07.007.

[29] Suganuma T, Workman JL. Signals and combinatorial functions of histone modifications. Annual Reviews in Biochemistry. 2011;80:473-99. DOI:

10.1146/annurev-biochem-061809-175347.

[30] Escobar TM, Loyola A, Reinberg D. Parental nucleosome segregation and the inheritance of cellular identity. Nature Review Genetics. 2021. DOI: 10.1038/s41576-020-00312-w.

[31] Bannister AJ, Kouzarides T. Regulation of chromatin by histone modifications. Cell Research. 2011;21 (3):381-95. DOI: 10.1038/cr.2011.22.

[32] Dykes IM, Emanueli C. Transcriptional and Post-transcriptional Gene Regulation by Long Non-coding RNA. Genomics Proteomics Bioinformatics. 2017;15(3):177-186. DOI: 10.1016/j.gpb.2016.12.005.

[33] Lim LP, Lau NC, Garrett-Engele P, Grimson A, Schelter JM, Castle J, Bartel DP, Linsley PS, Johnson JM. Microarray analysis shows that some microRNAs downregulate large numbers of target mRNAs. Nature. 2005;17;433(7027):769-73. DOI: 10.1038/nature03315.

[34] Valencia-Sanchez MA, Liu J, Hannon GJ, Parker R. Control of translation and mRNA degradation by miRNAs and siRNAs. Genes and Development. 2006;1;20(5):515-24. DOI: 10.1101/gad.1399806.

[35] Wang Y, Wang Z. Efficient back splicing produces translatable circular mRNAs. RNA. 2015;21(2):172-9. DOI: 10.1261/rna.048272.114.

[36] Zhou WY, Cai ZR, Liu J, Wang DS, Ju HQ, Xu RH. Circular RNA: metabolism, functions and interactions with proteins. Molecular Cancer. 2020; 14;19(1):172. DOI: 10.1186/s12943-020-01286-3.

[37] Chédin F. The DNMT3 family of mammalian de novo DNA methyltransferases. Progress in Molecular Biology and Translational Science. 2011;101:255-85. DOI: 10.1016/B978-0-12-387685-0.00007-X.

[38] Wu X, Zhang Y. TET-mediated active DNA demethylation: mechanism, function and beyond. Nature Review Genetics. 2017 Sep;18(9):517-534. DOI: 10.1038/nrg.2017.33.

[39] Morgan HD, Dean W, Coker HA, Reik W, Petersen-Mahrt SK. Activation-induced cytidine deaminase deaminates 5-methylcytosine in DNA and is expressed in pluripotent tissues: implications for epigenetic reprogramming. The Journal of Biological Chemistry. 2004;10;279(50): 52353-60. DOI: 10.1074/jbc.M407695200.

[40] Abdolmaleky HM, Cheng KH, Russo A, Smith CL, Faraone SV, Wilcox M, Shafa R, Glatt SJ, Nguyen G, Ponte JF, Thiagalingam S, Tsuang MT. Hypermethylation of the reelin (RELN) promoter in the brain of schizophrenic patients: a preliminary report. American Journal of Medical Genetics, Part B, Neuropsychiatric Genetics. 2005;5;134B (1):60-6. DOI: 10.1002/ajmg.b.30140.

[41] Yoshino Y, Kawabe K, Mori T, Mori Y, Yamazaki K, Numata S, Nakata S, Yoshida T, Iga J, Ohmori T, Ueno S. Low methylation rates of dopamine receptor D2 gene promoter sites in Japanese schizophrenia subjects. World Journal of Biological Psychiatry. 2016;17(6):449-56. DOI: 10.1080/15622975.2016.1197424.

[42] Huang HS, Akbarian S. GAD1 mRNA expression and DNA methylation in prefrontal cortex of subjects with schizophrenia. PLoS One. 2007;29;2(8):e809. DOI: 10.1371/journal.pone.0000809.

[43] Kordi-Tamandani DM, Dahmardeh N, Torkamanzehi A. Evaluation of hypermethylation and expression pattern of GMR2, GMR5, GMR8, and GRIA3 in patients with

schizophrenia. Gene. 2013;15;515(1): 163-6. DOI: 10.1016/j.gene.2012.10.075.

[44] Carrard A, Salzmann A, Malafosse A, Karege F. Increased DNA methylation status of the serotonin receptor 5HTR1A gene promoter in schizophrenia and bipolar disorder. Journal of Affective Disorders. 2011;132(3):450-3. DOI: 10.1016/j.jad.2011.03.018.

[45] Autry AE, Monteggia LM. Brain-derived neurotrophic factor and neuropsychiatric disorders. Pharmacological Reviews. 2012;64(2): 238-58. DOI: 10.1124/pr.111.005108.

[46] Kordi-Tamandani DM, Sahranavard R, Torkamanzehi A. DNA methylation and expression profiles of the brain-derived neurotrophic factor (BDNF) and dopamine transporter (DAT1) genes in patients with schizophrenia. Molecular Biology Reports. 2012;39(12):10889-93. DOI: 10.1007/s11033-012-1986-0.

[47] Ikegame T, Bundo M, Murata Y, Kasai K, Kato T, Iwamoto K. DNA methylation of the BDNF gene and its relevance to psychiatric disorders. Journal of Human Genetics. 2013;58(7): 434-8. DOI: 10.1038/jhg.2013.65.

[48] Çöpoğlu ÜS, Igci M, Bozgeyik E, Kokaçya MH, İğci YZ, Dokuyucu R, Ari M, Savaş HA. DNA Methylation of BDNF Gene in Schizophrenia. Medical Science Monitor. 2016;6;22:397-402. DOI: 10.12659/msm.895896.

[49] Mill J, Tang T, Kaminsky Z, Khare T, Yazdanpanah S, Bouchard L, Jia P, Assadzadeh A, Flanagan J, Schumacher A, Wang SC, Petronis A. Epigenomic profiling reveals DNA-methylation changes associated with major psychosis. American Journal of Human Genetics. 2008;82(3):696-711. DOI: 10.1016/j.ajhg.2008.01.008.

[50] Pries L, Gülöksüz S, Kenis G. DNA Methylation in Schizophrenia. Neuroepigenomics in Aging and Disease. Advances in Experimental Medicine and Biology, Vol. 978). https://doi.org/10.1007/978-3-319-53889-1_12

[51] Abdolmaleky HM, Cheng KH, Faraone SV, Wilcox M, Glatt SJ, Gao F, Smith CL, Shafa R, Aeali B, Carnevale J, Pan H, Papageorgis P, Ponte JF, Sivaraman V, Tsuang MT, Thiagalingam S. Hypomethylation of MB-COMT promoter is a major risk factor for schizophrenia and bipolar disorder. Human Molecular Genetics. 2006;1;15 (21):3132-45. DOI: 10.1093/hmg/ddl253.

[52] Aberg KA, McClay JL, Nerella S, Clark S, Kumar G, Chen W, Khachane AN, Xie L, Hudson A, Gao G, Harada A, Hultman CM, Sullivan PF, Magnusson PK, van den Oord EJ. Methylome-wide association study of schizophrenia: identifying blood biomarker signatures of environmental insults. JAMA Psychiatry. 2014;71(3): 255-64. DOI: 10.1001/jamapsychiatry.2013.3730.

[53] Kundakovic M, Gudsnuk K, Herbstman JB, Tang D, Perera FP, Champagne FA. DNA methylation of BDNF as a biomarker of early-life adversity. Proc Natl Acad Sci U S A. 2015;2;112(22):6807-13. DOI: 10.1073/pnas.1408355111.

[54] Hannon E, Dempster E, Viana J, Burrage J, Smith AR, Macdonald R, St Clair D, Mustard C, Breen G, Therman S, Kaprio J, Toulopoulou T, Hulshoff Pol HE, Bohlken MM, Kahn RS, Nenadic I, Hultman CM, Murray RM, Collier DA, Bass N, Gurling H, McQuillin A, Schalkwyk L, Mill J. An integrated genetic-epigenetic analysis of schizophrenia: evidence for co-localization of genetic associations and differential DNA methylation. Genome Biology. 2016;30;17(1):176. DOI: 10.1186/s13059-016-1041-x.

[55] Network and Pathway Analysis Subgroup of Psychiatric Genomics

Consortium. Psychiatric genome-wide association study analyses implicate neuronal, immune and histone pathways. Nature Neuroscience. 2015;18 (2):199-209. DOI: 10.1038/nn.3922.

[56] Pidsley R, Viana J, Hannon E, Spiers H, Troakes C, Al-Saraj S, Mechawar N, Turecki G, Schalkwyk LC, Bray NJ, Mill J. Methylomic profiling of human brain tissue supports a neurodevelopmental origin for schizophrenia. Genome Biology. 2014;15 (10):483. DOI: 10.1186/s13059-014-0483-2.

[57] Liu J, Chen J, Ehrlich S, Walton E, White T, Perrone-Bizzozero N, Bustillo J, Turner JA, Calhoun VD. Methylation patterns in whole blood correlate with symptoms in schizophrenia patients. Schizophrenia Bulletin. 2014;40(4):769-76. DOI: 10.1093/schbul/sbt080.

[58] Bönsch D, Wunschel M, Lenz B, Janssen G, Weisbrod M, Sauer H. Methylation matters? Decreased methylation status of genomic DNA in the blood of schizophrenic twins. Psychiatry Research. 2012;15;198(3): 533-7. DOI: 10.1016/j.psychres.2011.09.004.

[59] Melas PA, Rogdaki M, Ösby U, Schalling M, Lavebratt C, Ekström TJ. Epigenetic aberrations in leukocytes of patients with schizophrenia: association of global DNA methylation with antipsychotic drug treatment and disease onset. FASEB Journal. 2012;26 (6):2712-8. DOI: 10.1096/fj.11-202069.

[60] Bromberg A, Levine J, Nemetz B, Belmaker RH, Agam G. No association between global leukocyte DNA methylation and homocysteine levels in schizophrenia patients. Schizophrenia Research. 2008;101(1-3):50-7. doi: 10.1016/j.schres.2008.01.009.

[61] Veldic M, Guidotti A, Maloku E, Davis JM, Costa E. In psychosis, cortical interneurons overexpress DNA-methyltransferase 1. Proceedings of the National Academy of Sciences of the United States of America. 2005;8;102 (6):2152-7. DOI: 10.1073/pnas.0409665102.

[62] Kundakovic M, Chen Y, Costa E, Grayson DR. DNA methyltransferase inhibitors coordinately induce expression of the human reelin and glutamic acid decarboxylase 67 genes. Molecular Pharmacology. 2007;71(3): 644-53. DOI: 10.1124/mol.106.030635.

[63] Kundakovic M, Chen Y, Guidotti A, Grayson DR. The reelin and GAD67 promoters are activated by epigenetic drugs that facilitate the disruption of local repressor complexes. Molecular Pharmacology. 2009;75(2):342-54. DOI: 10.1124/mol.108.051763.

[64] Dong E, Ruzicka WB, Grayson DR, Guidotti A. DNA-methyltransferase1 (DNMT1) binding to CpG rich GABAergic and BDNF promoters is increased in the brain of schizophrenia and bipolar disorder patients. Schizophrenia Research. 2015;167(1-3): 35-41. DOI: 10.1016/j.schres.2014.10.030.

[65] Zhubi A, Veldic M, Puri NV, Kadriu B, Caruncho H, Loza I, Sershen H, Lajtha A, Smith RC, Guidotti A, Davis JM, Costa E. An upregulation of DNA-methyltransferase 1 and 3a expressed in telencephalic GABAergic neurons of schizophrenia patients is also detected in peripheral blood lymphocytes. Schizophrenia Research. 2009;111(1-3):115-22. DOI: 10.1016/j.schres.2009.03.020.

[66] Matrisciano F, Tueting P, Dalal I, Kadriu B, Grayson DR, Davis JM, Nicoletti F, Guidotti A. Epigenetic modifications of GABAergic interneurons are associated with the schizophrenia-like phenotype induced by prenatal stress in mice. Neuropharmacology. 2013;68:184-94.

DOI: 10.1016/j.neuropharm.2012.04.013.

[67] Saradalekshmi KR, Neetha NV, Sathyan S, Nair IV, Nair CM, Banerjee M. DNA methyl transferase (DNMT) gene polymorphisms could be a primary event in epigenetic susceptibility to schizophrenia. PLoS One. 2014;23;9(5):e98182. DOI: 10.1371/journal.pone.0098182.

[68] Biniszkiewicz D, Gribnau J, Ramsahoye B, Gaudet F, Eggan K, Humpherys D, Mastrangelo MA, Jun Z, Walter J, Jaenisch R. Dnmt1 overexpression causes genomic hypermethylation, loss of imprinting, and embryonic lethality. Molecular and Cellular Biology. 2002;22 (7):2124-35. DOI: 10.1128/mcb.22.7.2124-2135.2002.

[69] Sen GL, Reuter JA, Webster DE, Zhu L, Khavari PA. DNMT1 maintains progenitor function in self-renewing somatic tissue. Nature. 2010;28;463 (7280):563-7. DOI: 10.1038/nature08683.

[70] D'Aiuto L, Di Maio R, Mohan KN, Minervini C, Saporiti F, Soreca I, Greenamyre JT, Chaillet JR. Mouse ES cells overexpressing DNMT1 produce abnormal neurons with upregulated NMDA/NR1 subunit. Differentiation. 2011;82(1):9-17. DOI: 10.1016/j.diff.2011.03.003.

[71] Borowczyk E, Mohan KN, D'Aiuto L, Cirio MC, Chaillet JR. Identification of a region of the DNMT1 methyltransferase that regulates the maintenance of genomic imprints. Proceedings of the National Academy of Sciences of the United States of America. 2009;8;106(49):20806-11. DOI: 10.1073/pnas.0905668106.

[72] Saxena S, Choudhury S, Mohan KN. Reproducible differentiation and characterization of neurons from mouse embryonic stem cells. MethodsX. 2020;22;7:101073. DOI: 10.1016/j.mex.2020.101073.

[73] Saxena S, Maroju PA, Choudhury S, Anne A, Mohan KN. Analysis of transcript levels of a few schizophrenia candidate genes in neurons from a transgenic mouse embryonic stem cell model overexpressing DNMT1. Gene. 2020;5;757:144934. DOI: 0.1016/j.gene.2020.144934.